HYPNOTISM

A Complete Manual on Hypnotism for the
Beginner Intermediate and Advanced Practitioner

(Learn Mind Control Techniques to Become a
Master of Your Life)

Jose Frost

Published by Phil Dawson

Jose Frost

All Rights Reserved

Hypnotism: A Complete Manual on Hypnotism for the
Beginner Intermediate and Advanced Practitioner (Learn
Mind Control Techniques to Become a Master of Your Life)

ISBN 978-1-77485-367-2

Legal & Disclaimer

The information contained in this book is not designed to replace or take the place of any form of medicine or professional medical advice. The information in this book has been provided for educational and entertainment purposes only.

The information contained in this book has been compiled from sources deemed reliable, and it is accurate to the best of the Author's knowledge; however, the Author cannot guarantee its accuracy and validity and cannot be held liable for any errors or omissions. Changes are periodically made to this book. You must consult your doctor or get professional medical advice before using any of the suggested remedies, techniques, or information in this book.

Upon using the information contained in this book, you agree to hold harmless the Author from and against any damages, costs, and expenses, including any legal fees potentially resulting from the application of any of the information provided by this guide. This disclaimer applies to any damages or injury caused by the use and application, whether directly or indirectly, of any advice or information presented, whether for breach of contract, tort, negligence, personal injury, criminal intent, or under any other cause of action.

You agree to accept all risks of using the information presented inside this book. You need to consult a professional medical practitioner in order to ensure you are both able and healthy enough to participate in this program.

Table of Contents

Introduction

Hypnosis is the act of creating the state of mind that is altered, or consciousness. The use of hypnosis is widely employed in medical and psychiatric treatments. The term "hypnosis" is used to describe repetition of vocal commands and vocal suggestions that are delivered in a monotonous voice. The intention is to create a sense of calm and relaxation by focusing the mind to a specific topic or thought.

The most common usage of self-hypnosis is to assist a person to change their attitude and self-improvement. It is extremely beneficial for dealing with problems with anger, self-esteem issues, and self-confidence.

Self-hypnosis has been compared to surfing on a wave. When you spot an ocean wave, you can ride it and then steer your board. Surfers make use of the power of the waves to accomplish the feat. Once you have mastered the wave, you're at the top of the hill. It requires some time to master the art of surfing. One can get better and better with each practice. Self-hypnosis is a self-hypnosis technique. The same is true as you learn how to enter the hypnotic zone and learn to apply various methods to increase the ability of the mind.

Some people are not susceptible to hypnosis easily, but totally unhypnotizable people aren't there. Self-hypnosis is regarded as a weak self-hypnosis, however with it the possibility exists of energizing yourself to do many things.

Hypnosis is an unnatural state of the mind. A lot of people have been in a state of hypnosis without realizing that they were in it. For instance, if you're all your attention on something that you do not know anything else at that moment in time then you're in an hypnotic state.

The essence of hypnosis is having an focused attention on a specific subject , and not allowing for other activities. It is said that hypnosis functions like a light beam that lets you access the mental resources. Through hypnosis training the person is in a position to trigger different areas of the mind to accomplish certain tasks.

Chapter 1: A More In-Depth Analyse Of Hypnosis

Hypnosis can be described as a state of Trance that is marked with intense relaxation sexiness and heightened imagination. In a state of hypnosis it's not like you're asleep because although internally you're aware, you're not fully aware.

If you induce someone to hypnotize them to do so, they are experiencing a kind of dreaming. The person is aware and alert however, they are unable to focus on all the distractions within the environment. In simple terms, it can cause an individual to be focused on the things the person hypnotizing them.

If you've ever had a daydream feeling lost and completely lost in the dream, where you didn't pay attention to or pay any focus on what was happening around you, then you'll learn more about how hypnosis affects you.

Hypnosis helps the world of the mind seem real to the subject mostly because it completely engages the subject's emotions. The imaginary scenarios could trigger emotions like sadness, happiness or fear, and other feelings. If you're engaging someone in hypnosis, they may even start to shiver in his/her seat when they feel shocked or scared by something.

Based on Milton Erickson, one of the most famous experts in the art of hypnotism. We all are hypnotized at some point or another throughout our daily lives. But, the majority of psychiatrists view real hypnosis to be a kind of trance that is often brought on through deliberate concentration as well as relaxation exercise. The state of deep hypnosis is similar to the tranquil state of mind you feel between wakefulness and sleep.

In a normal hypnosis session, the person adheres to the advice of their hypnotist, or even his own to make they appear to be real. For example the hypnotist telling the person that their leg has increased to the size it is, in reality, the person will think and feel that his leg is swelling and getting larger than it was before. If a hypnotist says that the subject has eaten something that is sour, the person will likely experience the sensation of tanginess inside his mouth. Even though the person is aware that the image is not real, he is unable to not help but think and feel about what the hypnotist is suggesting.

The trance-like experience makes the person feel relaxed at peace, calm, and free of inhibition. The reason for this is that the hypnotists help the subject tune out any worries anxiety, anxieties, and fears which normally allow a person control over their actions. The sensation of those who are in a hallucinogenic state is similar with the experience you get while watching a movie, and you become so absorbed in the plot that the worries you have about financial worries, family tensions and other concerns go away and you find yourself wondering what's going on in the movie.

In a state hypnosis, a person's mind is calm and highly susceptible to suggestion too. This means that , if the hypnotist demands the person to perform a task, the person will follow the instructions.

How Does Hypnosis Actually Work

Your mind operates in three different levels: subconscious conscious, unconscious, and subconscious. The conscious mind governs every action you take conscious. Your subconscious mind stores all your memories you've built up to this point. It is the the home to all of your memories from the past and helps to facilitate the communication between the conscious and subconscious minds by storing the information in your subconscious mind, so that anything you do is guided by your subconscious mind using the information that is retrieved from the subconscious mind.

The subconscious mind is connected to a vast information storage and that's why it assists you in thinking about things, think through issues, and take decisions. It develops ideas and plans and then entrusts your conscious mind with the task of executing them.

When you are suddenly thinking about something, you've already considered it in your subconscious mind. It also controls our actions automatically, like walking, breathing or driving. The conscious mind functions as the primary driver behind all of the actions we carry out.

While we're awake, our conscious brain is at work to assess our thoughts so it is able to make choices. Furthermore it processes information and transmits this information back to the unconscious mind. When we asleep, our conscious mind is asleep and the subconscious mind takes over and is in completely in control.

Relaxation exercises and focusing (they are a part of the hypnosis procedure) help to calm our mind to make it less active while we are thinking. This is the reason why, when we are in hypnosis, even if the subject is awake the subject isn't concerned about worries and anxiety of making a mistake. The hypnotist is able to connect directly to your subconscious. Since your subconscious mind is in control of your body you're relaxed and more creative than before because the mind of your conscious filters every bit of information you take in and allows it to flow easily.

If the conscious mind doesn't transmit its thoughts and process the info it receives the subject is able to feel like the suggestions made by the hypnotist originate from their own subconscious in the first place, rather than from a different person. The person who is hypnotized immediately and instantly responds to these suggestions in the same manner as the way he or she would react to own thoughts. But, because the subconscious mind is an instinct to survive, its own beliefs and conscience it is unlikely that the subject will be able to accept everything that the hypnotist suggests.

The subconscious mind is also responsible for bodily sensations such as emotions and emotional feelings, touch tasting, and sight this is why, in the event that the unconscious mind becomes opened the hypnotist is able to communicate with it and initiate all the different emotions. This is why the hypnotized person is able to feel and taste various items when they are in the state of trance. If a person is in a state of suggestion the hypnotist is also able to make up false memories and experiences.

This is how hypnosis operates and how hypnotists are able to influence and control those in their Trance. If you can learn to hypnotize people, you will be able to influence them, control them, and influence them to do what you want.

For example, if you don't want your spouse to behave in a particular way or take a particular decision that impacts you, you could enter into the mind of your partner and make them think differently, by manipulating the subconscious mind. In the same way, if you want employees to act exactly what you tell them to do and be productive so that you can accomplish your objectives You can use hypnosis to influence them and make them perform their tasks effectively and follow your directions.

If you can use hypnosis to your advantage it is possible to influence any person. Be aware that each of us has our own conscience as well as a set of values. So, you can't direct someone to perform things that are not right or that the person in hypnosis might find inappropriate and inconvenient because if you offer an unpalatable suggestion, you could rouse people from their state of trance. The person might not be able to trust you again.

After we've gone over the basics of hypnosis the next chapter in which you will be taught how to use hypnosis to influence anyone.

Chapter 2: Self-hypnosis for Motivation and achieving Success

Motivation is among the main reason why we aren't being successful. The lack of motivation we experience is often triggered by our preconceived ideas and thoughts such as fear of failure, discomfort with a task , or something else.

These preconceived notions are imbedded in our minds, and create seemingly unsurmountable obstacles in the way of motivation finding it's way to our daily lives. This means that our minds have been trained to be averse to our needs and desires , instead of working towards our own success.

The voice that is in our minds becomes our biggest critic, as well as a negative influence, generating negative thoughts that constantly tell us to not do something for a variety of insignificant motives. Self-hypnosis, too, can prove to be a huge help.

Self-hypnosis is a method to guide our minds to transform negative experiences to positive ones, so that our minds are in sync with our daily life, instead of battling against it. By using self-hypnosis you can teach your brain to be positive in the face of adversity and difficulties, which ultimately, increases motivation. Before this, let's test to understand the absence of motivation.

Evidence of Lack of Motivation

It is essential to note that in this book, we're not discussing the absence of motivation to wash your vehicle on Sunday morning , or doing other chores around and around your home. This book is about that part of motivation, which if not in adequate amounts can negatively impact your work, personal, and relationships, and eventually it can cause anxiety and depression.

However, it's crucial to keep in mind that if the inability to complete the first kind of job (the routine and sometimes the tedious chores) remains unresolved for a long time after which it may turn into a loss of motivation to live the life.

You must be aware of this aspect and get taking on the tedious but vital chores as well. There are certain indicators which will let you know loud and loud that you are lacking motivation:

• Losing interest in everything you do.

* Delaying important work assignments and other tasks.

* Not being able to finish tasks in a timely manner.

You may lose track of your life's purpose and objectives.

Feeling a sense inadequacy.

Feeling depressed or depressed.

How to Make Use of Self-Hypnosis for Motivation

You can make use of this technique in order to change your negative thoughts to positive ones that keep your energy levels up and keep you on the right path to accomplish your goals. Use these tips:

* Lay or sit in a relaxedand comfortable place.

Shut your eyes, and concentrate on your breathing for a few seconds until you are completely relaxed and at ease.

Imagine yourself in a hall standing in the front of an escalator that is moving in a downward direction.

Be aware of the movement of the escalator as well as all the other details surrounding it. Be aware of the steps that appear to move downwards. Pay attention to the handles either sideof you, and can secure yourself to ensure your security.

Imagine slowly yourself getting on the escalator and then slowly moving towards the downwards. Relax every time the escalator gently moves down.

* As you begin to fall make yourself aware that it is time to increase your motivation levels to ensure that you are able to achieve your objectives.

Be confident and affirm that you have were always aware that the right time to realize your self and become self-actualized will be in your life, and this small activity is the very first thing you can do to that goal.

You should tell yourself it's time for you to be in control of your life is now and you're ready for it.

* You've arrived at the top of the ascender. Imagine a large, wide and bright room. There is a most loved chair at one end in the space. Take a seat on the chair and close your eyes.

* Relax as much as you can on your comfy chair.

Think about the goal you wish to achieve and imagine yourself reaching the goal successfully. Imagine a vivid scene what happens when you accomplish your goal. Include what you experience, feel, smell as well as other sensations.

In your mind, take a moment to think about the very first step you took toward generating motivation to accomplish your goals. Remind yourself how easy to obtain the things you want, as long as you truly desire it.

Keep in mind that the most difficult part of reaching your goal is getting to where you want to be. Once you've taken that first move, everything falls into the right place.

Finding the motivation to complete the next step is simple due to the success of the first and so on. Every step you take toward your goals, you'll discover the path getting more free of obstacles and difficulties to keep your motivation up.

While you are soaking in the bliss of self-hypnosis Repetition the following motivation-building ideas to your self:

* I am determined to conquer challenges and move forward on the road to success.

* Fear is nothing more than an emotion and does not have any influence over me.

* I am energized and determined to do whatever that is required to be successful.

* I am adamant and determination to turn my visions into reality.

Each step I take toward my goals gives me incentive to move on to another step.

Remember that you are the only one who can have control over your life and happenings. So, get in the wheel and drive wherever your heart and your mind desire to lead you. Therefore, follow your dreams and don't let the absence of motivation to impede your advancement.

Chapter 3: The Way to Engage in Conversational Hypnosis

There is no need to be prepared to perform "Conversational Hypnosis" or understand how to use self hypnosis. Through taking a few deep breaths through your mouth and letting air flow out gently and slowly out of your nostrils, simply let it go.

Your jaw and shoulders should be relaxed . As you stretch your fingers to your arms you will feel the softening of your hands. Allow it to flow through all of you i.e. through your back, chest and legs. It should also go all the way to your toes. When compared to other people you, take note that your hands might feel warmer.

Here's the list of a few things you must do when performing hypnosis:

21

To get rid of a particular habit, such as smoking or drinking, the person should have usually agreed to the session. To first inform the person whom you're talking to about the things that make her unhappy You must be a calm listener, and you must be able to listen to the person. To entice targets to do something they wouldn't otherwise do the use of conversational hypnosis to induce people who do not even realize of the fact that they're being at the mercy of hypnosis.

Get the attention of your target, and make sure it is in good standing. Following the completion of the first step , since the target is now aware that you're eager to address her problems and want to assist her to solve her problems, you can accomplish this. Let the person you are helping feel at ease with you and your team. Do not try to be authoritative in your voice and make sure you use soft words.

Create rapport with your desired target. Rapport is about getting your subject engaged with your conversation so that they believe it can be helpful to her and can be exciting to her. Establishing a strong rapport is crucial prior to beginning and delivering the real message that is the basis of the hypnotic conversation. The person you are targeting should be interested in the message you are saying and be remain secure.

Try to induce the target into sleep. To induce a state insanity where the person has fallen into a routine of agreeing to what you say and make admiring suggestions to which the target accepts. In relation to the issues the person is in the statements must be closely correlated to allow her to easily relate to what is experiencing and also what is being stated.

Make your suggestions known to the person in question. Slowly and gradually inculcating the mind of the target that you would like to share and wish her in her unconscious mind to accept as true that is when you start the actual illusion of hypnosis. This will lead to get the person to translate those ideas into action and help is necessary to be successful.

Chapter 4: The Common Issues Which can be addressed when dealing with Hypnosis

Hypnosis is a solution to many various issues that we as human beings, have to deal with every day. In reality, there are some incredibly small issues that are not solved by the application of the hypnosis method. Many have discovered in the last two centuries, hypnosis can be an excellent method to alter the way you think, ease, or and reframe things that happened in your life or conditions that affect you, to allow you to transcend them and bring about peace and peace and. I'm sure you're seeking a way to make your life easier and happier, or else you would not have bought this book. To help you with that I've listed a few ways in which hypnosis may help ease various common ailments that sufferers face regularly. These are discussed in this section. You can use them yourself by recording recordings by yourself or with the assistance of a certified hypnotherapist.

Depression

Depression is a well-known ailment that many people throughout the world struggle with. It affects kids as young as 5 and in adults of all age groups. It can be debilitating and even life end if it is not dealt with properly. People who suffer from depression feel they are missing loved ones and family members because of their inability to get over the emotional turmoil they feel when in major depression phase.

The great thing is that hypnosis can be an excellent method to deal these problems. With hypnosis, one are able to begin experiencing the world more. You will be more secure and experience greater joy. Though depression is often linked by a chemical imbalance within the brain, depression is successfully treated using the power of hypnosis.

There are a variety of methods to utilize hypnosis to manage depression. One option is to utilize the hypnosis sessions to redefine the events of the individual's life that cause the most stress. This is an approach of reframe the circumstances, shifting the negative to an optimistic. Affirmations can be one method that can change the negative and turn them into something positive. These positive changes can be achieved using hypnosis , where you look into the past events and alter the way people view those experiences in a positive light and also aid them in realizing that they're not this person and that the events that occurred are no longer harmful to them.

Anxiety

Anxiety is another mental illness that many suffer from. It's also one that can be managed or cured by the method of applying a relaxation hypnosis method to assist the individual in getting past the anxiety and to the space that feels secure and at ease.

If people experience anxiety, it's usually because of a circumstance that occurred in their lives, which put them in a state of fight or flight. This is because they haven't learned to manage their fight or flight mode and, as a result, the body goes into this fear-based state in random situations which would not trigger this kind of reaction. This can lead to many issues within the life of a person. Anxiety can cause damage to relationships and the psychological state of the individual suffering from anxiety. People will encounter situations that trigger similar reactions and be anxious when the fear is unfounded. They will be unable to moving out of their homes and lead them to be denied job opportunities, getting to know new people, remaining in touch with family members or, sometimes, hinder the need to leave their home completely, which can lead to an even more severe disorder known as Agoraphobia.

Utilizing a technique of hypnosis known as relaxation, you will start to ease the symptoms that are associated with anxiety.

Begin by getting yourself as comfortable as is possible.

* You can lay down or recline in recliners in a comfortable position.

Begin to count down between 1 and 10 through your brain.

Breathing slowly in through your mouth and slowly via your nostrils.

Control your breathing and allow your breathing to become rhythmic, with four seconds between each intake and out-take of breath.

* As you breathe in, you should tighten up your muscles throughout your body.

Inhale and let your muscles relax in your body.

* Use a soft tone to talk to yourself and to make affirmative and positive statements which will help you to achieve a more peaceful and relaxed mindset.

Example: "I am safe and safe in this location."

Mindset issues

Many suffer from mental problems with their mindset. This could be due to misinformation our families have instilled into our minds since we were young. They could also be the things we have observed from people around us that have been ingrained in us and caused anxiety, fear, or negative reactions within us. Mindset is a way of defining the person we are and the values we hold. It can be a source of strength or weakness. If, for instance, you're always told you're not worthy of love, when you get the chance to experience genuine love, you'll hinder it due to the notions that were instilled into you from a young time. This is the reason it is crucial to address the issues of mindset and develop an optimistic mindset in yourself.

Once you have begun to shift your perspective, you will be able to begin making positive choices and improvements in your life. If you don't have positive thoughts and feelings then you are bound to continue to suffer unhappy and disappointed. You'll notice patterns that allow you to focus on the negative aspects of life, and it will result in an unending cycle of negativity that is preventing your ability to see the positive aspects of life.

Hypnosis can aid in all of these. With the positive power of affirmations you could employ the same strategy as previously mentioned for anxiety relief, however instead of phrase, "I am safe and secure in this location," you would use an affirmation positive which will allow you to reframe your thoughts and make more positive connections inside your mind.

The bridges you'll create will ease the burden of feeling unworthy and assist you in understanding that you're worthy of good things happening in your world.

A number of affirmations can be usedto:

"I deserve the greatest things in my life."

"Everything me do has been fantastic."

"I make magic through my words."

"I am a magnet for money."

"I I am beloved by plenty of people."

Smoking cessation

Many people begin smoking in their teens due to either trying to appear cool with their peers and friends or to escape from family drama which turned their lives upside down. Smoking is the most common cause of death in the US alone , and should be treated as a toxins However, a lot of people are suffering daily from their attempts to quit smoking. There are a few people who quit smoking without problems. But, they are very few and far between. If you are unable to stop smoking, there's the option of hypnotherapy. Hypnotherapy uses using hypnosis in order to change the behaviour that you would like to alter.

If you smoke for prolonged durations it will cause your body to depend on this substance to live and function at its fullest. This can lead to an addiction that affects the mind and triggers your mind to want smoking cigarettes even at the least inconvenient moments. If you've ever seen ads that promote not smoking, then you've certainly witnessed the power smoking cigarettes will exert on you. If you're smokers, you might not be aware of how enslaving smoking is until you realize the perspective from outside your box. Because smoking cigarettes is addicting and addictive it can be very difficult to get people to quit smoking. This is where hypnosis can prove useful. Utilizing a hypnosis method known as smoking cessation, can cleanse out the toxins in your body subconsciously manner and produce an even stronger cutting experience from the addiction to smoking. There are many techniques or sessions that could be employed to stop smoking cigarettes, and as an accredited hypnotherapist I suggest you find the most appropriate one for your needs , and then utilizing it repeatedly for several weeks until you are no longer feeling smoking cigarettes so powerful. After proper application of these techniques it is possible to break your addiction to smoking in just 8 weeks of regular use of hypnosis.

Weight loss

Statistics show that America is obese, far more than any other nation. This is a huge threat for the overall health of our nation and to the overall health of residents of the nation. As a proponent of an ideal weight I am aware that hypnosis is an excellent option to reverse these trends and put the American people in a more positive mindset. Through modifying your eating habits and the triggers for overeating and eating habits, you can start to alter your diet and weight.

The most important reason overweight people are because of emotional eating. Children are taught to eat our food at dinner time, even when we're satisfied. Also, we are taught to fill our bodies with sweets and ice cream when we feel blue either celebrating or just watching a film. This leads to eating too much. Overeating means eating more than we really need. For some it's unhealthy food items, sugary drinks snacks, foods high in fat like beef, pork, chicken, as well as processed foods that offer zero nutritional value.

With the help of behavioral modifications using behavior modification, you can create plans to alter how you think about food and organize your meals. It will be used in your hypnosis session to ensure that the changes are anchored in your mind, to ensure that you don't consume too much food or focus on eating more. It will stop your desire to eat to satisfy your emotional needs and will help you learn the proper behaviours that are associated with foods and food.

A few changes you could incorporate into the hypnosis session include:

"I do not need food to make me feel full."

"I consume only what I require to survive and not more."

"My feelings no longer dictate what I consume."

"When I'm feeling low I'll go for an outing."

"Food isn't a source of comfort."

Now that I've discussed the basics of hypnosis and the ways it can benefit the health of you as well, I'd like you to learn more about the essential steps you need to do to ensure that you are able to enjoy a safe use of the art of hypnosis. This book has been designed to assist you in not just master these methods for yourself , but also give you more understanding of what it can do for you. Next chapter I'll review the checklist of steps to follow in order for the best hypnosis experience. I will begin by assessing your ability to suggest and then move to the methods, the inductions, and the suggestions in the hypnosis system, as well as the techniques to modify forming and the methods to differentiate between how your body is interpreted by the people you are in hypnosis with.

Chapter 5: Self-hypnosis

Self-hypnosis can be described as an act of self-control, and it is employed to control your thoughts, desires and desires. It is usually thought to be more challenging than hypnosis and requires much more discipline and discipline. Self-hypnosis is an effective technique for combating negative emotions that arise from certain situations and events, by channeling them towards the right direction, towards positive thinking. As we've seen with the example that of Gary (our PTSD combat veteran) that it is possible to look at a painful experience and gain insight from it by looking at it from a different perspective. This method is applicable to self-hypnosis as well, and can be used to address anything from stress, low concentration and difficulties sleeping. Self-hypnosis isn't a good life-saving tool if you're capable of sustaining the kind of discipline needed to use it, and, consequently, gain from it.

Self-hypnosis to achieve success

Self-hypnosis can be described as a method of dealing with the functions of your mind through opening your mind to different perspectives on an array of issues or challenges, as well as events. The subconscious mind functions independently. It doesn't make a sudden decision that it's time to quit breathing, or cease your heartbeat. The subconscious isn't wired in this way. It's programmed to constantly be working, storing the information you do not need in the present Sorting through your memories, processing subtexts and meaning, and maintaining all essential functions of your body.

Self-hypnosis allows you to unlock the immense potential that your unconscious mind holds the main factor. It can help you to train your mind to make everything easy, be it breaking a habit, achieving better results on the job, or being more comfortable in your interactions with other people. It can aid in the removal of the creative blockages, stage fright and anxiety, and can even aid you in losing weight. In essence, self-hypnosis can be employed to conquer all challenges that you may face.

Self-hypnosis can help you get rid of mental obstacles that block your way of reaching the goals you've set to achieve. The blocks you encounter can be traced to your own conscious mental state and the way it interprets how you see yourself. Self-perception could result from any of a range of causes, such as the fact that you allow others to decide on your behalf on what your capabilities are. Self-hypnosis is a method to teach you how to break through mental blockages within the conscious mind to shift your beliefs and self-assertions that hinder your progress in your daily life. Your subconscious mind is constantly adept at what it is programmed to accomplish. If you can program it to perform the actions you want to do, you'll succeed in achieving that need. If you notice dust falling into your eyes, it's the conscious part of your brain that is be curious about what's falling, but it's the unconscious mind that instantly closes your eyes , thereby protecting your eyes from dust. Your conscious brain is what that creates issues, while the unconscious mind is the brain's mainstay and will ensure that you don't waste the remainder of the day trying to wash grit out of your eyes. Through letting yourself be a part of your subconscious mind, you'll create a bridge between your conscious mind so that you can bring all your imaginative innovative, imaginative and adventurous thoughts and actions to the next level. Through this process you'll discover who you are and what you're able to do. Self-hypnosis can help you manage your life and live the life you've always wanted through helping you overcome your own limitations. You are the most significant obstacle to overcome. When you tap into your subconscious, you will be able to effectively remove yourself from the way you are.

The definition of success isn't just about money or fame. For some, getting it through the day without succumbing to anxiety, mood swings or other conflicts is a sign of success. Others, it's getting the respect they deserve. These things usually require a certain level confidence and belief that you can achieve your goals that you've set for yourself. If you're someone who is doubting yourself using self-hypnosis, it can be a great tool to uncover confidence in themselves that they never believed they could ever attain. Self-hypnosis lets you offer yourself the gift of confidence and belief that you are able to achieve your goals and aspirations. Change the way that you speak to yourself about your capabilities and potential, and reprogramming your self-image from a negative one to make it positive, you will be able to unlock talents and talents you might not thought you had. In exposing yourself to the unconscious reality of who you really are and what you're able to do is the way to live an enriched life.

How does self-hypnosis work?

All the things you think, feel or do is stored in your subconscious. Within these thoughts and emotions are the negative thoughts that you hold about yourself. The way you first feel about an event can greatly influence how you will react to the same situation or feeling later on. Self-hypnosis can be a method of changing your emotional reactions to stop them from affecting your life, through confronting your triggers and assisting you to learn from your previous experiences. We decide how we respond to situations and even though many people aren't convinced that it's true It is in our own control to decide on the appropriate response to situations that cause us to display anger or fear, resentment, or jealousy. The negative feelings can manifest into negative behavior that is reflected on us and could affect our performance in all aspects that we live in. Finding the root of them all is a self-hypnosis technique that could be the best friend you have.

You are in control of not just your reactions to situations that trigger unacceptable behavior, but you can also control your perception of your self as person. What drives every word you speak and act is the way in which you view yourself. Are you satisfied with your self-esteem? Do you have faith in yourself? It is possible that you believe in yourself but is that a true answer to these questions? Truthfully, the majority of humans are plagued by doubt. In some instances this doubt could be crippling and stop us from being the best we could be.

A classic self-hypnosis session comprises three elements. The three parts must be performed in the exact order as described in order to be successful. As with all procedures it is recommended to be familiar with the stages prior to attempting the actual procedure. The first step is to prepare for a self-hypnosis session and the next stage involves the actual process of hypnosis. Thirdly, the final stage concerns the precautions that should be taken as well as how to conclude the session.

Part 1 Part 1 - Preparation

The first part of the session should be easy. It will make sure that you don't diverge from the desired outcome of using self-hypnosis. A complicated beginning can create confusion and you could get out of your way spending time in a useless session. The preparation of the self-hypnosis session is a series of elements that must be considered prior to the second phase can be initiated. Let's take a look at these aspects in greater detail.

Place

Self-hypnosis usually takes place in the privacy of a space. The location you select is vital, since it determines the mood. The type of setting you're in prior to initiating self-hypnosis can have an impact on your thinking. You must be in the quiet of the room, and be in a location with a minimal amount of noise and a small chance of disturbance. Talking or walking around can add noise during a hypnosis session. Make sure the space is comfortable, not too cold or hot. It has also been proven that soft lighting can be beneficial and creates a more effective self-hypnosis space.

Temperature

As we mentioned before The temperature of the room is vital. In a room that is extremely hot, it will cause you to sweat and make you be uncomfortable.

Additionally, there's also the possibility of being dehydrated due to excessive sweating. A cold space however can affect circulation of blood within your body, and could make you forget about the relaxation session. It is therefore recommended to select the temperature that's not too hot nor too cold. If you are planning to be sitting for long periods of time during your session it is crucial.

Clothing

Do not wear tight-fitting clothing. They can distract you from your session as it could make you uncomfortable while sitting for prolonged periods. Simple, loose clothing is the preferred choice. Shorts, sweats or loose shirts are ideal to wear to an hypnotic session with a self-hypnotherapist.

Solitude

The most significant danger to a session of self-hypnosis is distraction and disturbance from external sources. Before beginning a session, make sure that all phones are turned off, all windows are locked, doors shut, and alarm clocks are turned off. If you are able, inform your family members living with you to be still or to choose the time that they are not present or do not interrupt you. Don't begin the session if you are expecting to receive an important phone call. Complete the call and any other tasks before beginning the session. This session is only for you. Everyone else shouldn't be permitted to disrupt the session.

Posture

Posture is another important aspect of the art of hypnosis. Your posture is just as important as the place you are sitting. Select your favourite chairs or the most pleasurable seat within the room for your time. Make sure you are sitting straight, with your arms and legs uncrossed and comfortable. Leaning forward or slouching to the side isn't a good posture due to the fact that it could cause back pain due to the length of the exercise.

Agendas

Always prepare an agenda for your session. Don't begin your session thinking that you can just "wing" it. It is a process that is methodical. It is therefore essential to be prepared with a plan prior to beginning. Your agenda may be as simple as you want. For some it might be a way to relax. Others may be to tackle the emotional stress of a situation or another challenge. If you don't decide on an agenda that you can focus on, your brain isn't able to concentrate. What's the purpose behind this? Answer the question in full and then choose whom you will respond to your reason for conducting the self-hypnosis process.

Here are some goals for a session of self-hypnosis:

O Eliminating bad habits. If it's drinking too much or drug use or an overeating habit the use of hypnosis is used to get rid of these vices.

A boost of brain functions is the most common reason to begin engaging in self-hypnosis for a regular exercise. It is a brain organ which could be trained to perform the way you wish it to. If you can train it to think fast and rationally it will. Self-hypnosis can assist you in gaining control over how your brain processes information and stores it.

O The peace of mind is something that everyone wants in this day and age. Many people lead such hectic lives that they seldom achieve peace. Self-hypnosis helps them reach an euphoriac state. Like meditation, the results of self-hypnosis can be felt even when they are not in the middle of a session. The goal is to reach the root of what's that is bothering you and then experience relief.

The initial stage of self-hypnosis is to prepare yourself mentally and physically. This step is of the utmost importance. Make sure that you've done the right thing to establish the ideal conditions for self-hypnosis to be successful, by addressing the factors that are listed above. Every solid structure needs an underlying foundation. The first step is the basis of a properly-structured self-hypnosis experience. Once we've created the stage and ensured that we're in a calm setting, that reduces the possibility of being disturbed or interrupted, let's think about the session it's own.

Part 2 Induction

The second phase of the session examines the actual beginning of self-hypnosis, and the importance of ensuring that the process of induction takes place gradually and carefully. A quick start to the session may hinder its success in the end

Therefore, it is of vital importance to take particular note of the information below.

Close your eyes

Closing your eyes can have the effect of calming and tends to bring the environment down. Closing your eyes symbolizes of closing your eyes to the world because our eyes are the first thing we use to view and communicate with ahead of all other sensory. Closing your eyes can help minimize the visual distractions created by your surroundings. Nearly half of distracting factors can be avoided simply with closing the eyes. This will also reduce the amount of light entering your eyes.

Restricting your thoughts

This is the most important aspect during the entire session. Before you begin your session, it's crucial to not allow any unintentional thoughts to take you off the path during your session. They can cause distraction and can cause you to drift away from the goal that the sessions are intended to achieve. But, it's not simple to keep your mind free of thoughts. When you first begin self-hypnosis, you'll be able to see more than a dozen thoughts wandering in and out of your head. What's the menu for dinner? Did I forget to leave the iron connected? Don't get discouraged. It requires practice to eliminate any competing thoughts. If you keep practicing, you will eventually master the ability to wander off from your goal. When you've successfully eliminated any thoughts that are not yours then you are able to move on to the next phase of your practice.

Integrity

The best way to deal with thoughts that you are incapable of removing from your mind is to think of you as an passive viewer, or a non-engaged observer instead of a participant. Be conscious of your thoughts, however, don't attach any significance or value to these thoughts. Your mind is just operating, just like it does every day. It is best to remain silent and let the thoughts flow instead of making mental comments or react or get frustrated by them. For instance, if your favourite food is the thought that is running through your head and you don't want to let it go, allow it to go. Do not let it influence your thoughts. Make sure to eat prior to a session to avoid the thoughts about food forming in your mind. It's also recommended to drink plenty of water in order to keep yourself hydrated however, not enough to stop your session to go to the restroom. Respect for your thoughts is a great way to stop your thoughts from becoming distracting.

Find tension points

The body is tense in various areas that need to be relaxed prior to begin your hypnosis process. You can identify each of these places in your body. To identify these spots you must be aware of the different tensions in each part of your body separately. Start with your feet and slowly move up toward your head. Concentrate on each area with a keen eye until you feel the tension go away. Imagine the tension disappearing from your body is an effective method to ease into relaxation. Visualizing the path it will take in its departure helps you to connect with the tension and let it go. The release of tension must be gradual and not rush because hurrying will defeat the point in the process.

Breathing

Breathing is an integral component of an hypnosis session for self. Breathing can aid in slowing down and relax to allow you to begin your session with a state of mind that's conducive for the session. (Slow deep breathing can also be beneficial for your health as an aside).

When you breathe your lung's lungs expand (inhalation) as well as contract (exhalation). Be aware of these changes. Imagine the breath flowing in the and from your lung. Slow breathing can help your mind to relax and become more focused. When you breathe in you will be able to visualize positive energy flowing into your body. When you exhale you can imagine the negative energy released by exhaling your breath. It is possible to make use of your imagination to imagine the energy flowing into and out of your body. Imagine it as a solid and giving inhalations and exhalations the appropriate colors to show their individual characteristics as positively or negatively. Whatever device you decide to use to improve your visualization the benefits of the practice of mindful, deep breathing is yours and only yours Choose a method that you like.

Imagine

Hypnosis is based on your imagination to bring you in a state of mind where your mind is at ease and focussed. When your mind is soaring and you're ready to relax completely. Make it appear as if you're on highest point of your favorite mountain, and nothing is beneath you. Now imagine you have the ability to fly, however, you haven't yet used it. Make a few steps towards the edge, then let go. Imagine falling and, as you begin to fall, you can feel yourself sliding before eventually being lifted. This is the beginning of your liberation from the mental fatigues of everyday life. Create your imagination as vivid as it can be. The more precise your imagination is the more difficult it is for your mind to believe it.

Delve deeper

After you've taken your first step of trust, it's time to dive deeper into your thoughts. When you're flying take a picture of a lake you could see from the mountain that you were standing on the top of or a meadow that is green. You can see it expanding as you get closer. Notice the sun's rays lighting the waters and the grasses that grow on the banks. Feel the breeze rushing by you and feel the feeling of flying. Draw the scene as you take off, making the experience appear as real as if you were watching the unfold in front of your eyes. You should be able manage your flight - speed and altitude. The gravity doesn't matter any more. You have control over everything.

Statements

This is the phase of self-hypnosis when you begin working toward your goal. Choose a phrase that will lead you to your desired purpose during the time. For instance, if your aim is to achieve greater success at work, your statement could read such as "Need for me to look outside of the box". For instance, you could say "I need to perform better in my work". Make the statements clear and precise. Make sure they don't be a way to ask questions like, "Should I perform better?" or "Maybe I ought to perform better". These kinds of statements let your mind to drift away from your goals, and can throw your objectives into doubt. The way you express it can have an impact. If your assertion is clear and clear the mind will take it as factual.

When you have reached the point where you feel as if you're floating, repeat the phrase in loop for a few minutes. Repeat the statement slowly 5 minutes at a time, with intervals between every repetition. After that, gradually increase the frequency until you say it 10 times in a minute, then 15 until you've reached 30 repetitions in a minute.

Chapter 6: Hypnotic Tests And Other Things You Need to Be Educated About

Okay, I know that I mentioned that this isn't a hypnosis-training manual, but I think I'd better include some suggestions for quick and instant hypnotic inductions , as and what do I mean by "not completely' hypnotic test. Let's begin by introducing these non-hypnotic methods. They're not hypnotic since they have more about the physiology of how the body works rather than the concept of hypnosis.

1)Hand Lock: Place your palms together and then interlock your fingers. Then, spread your elbows to ensure that your fingers remain locked, but your palms are not touching. While keeping your fingers locked extend your arms over your head. Try to break your hands. You'll find that you're not able to do it, as the muscles aren't pulling this way.

2.) Contact Fingers Place your palms on the same side and then interlock your fingers. Spread both index fingers and put your fingers in a cross. Expand your index fingers until they are just a few centimeters from each other at the tips : 1 to 2 centimeters is sufficient. Relax your eyes, and imagine "My fingers are drawn to one another" in a continuous manner. After a few minutes you will notice that your fingers be touching.

These tests are used to showing that people adhere to instructions and produce results that can be predicted beforehand. The next couple of tricks can be somewhat hypnotic as a result of the language employed, but don't require an euphoria, though some could be used to induce just by adding the words "and put your head down... then then sleep" when the test was to be successful. These are tricks you can ask your entire audience to do following your talk to ensure that they are willing to listen to your advice and convince them that they could be willing participants in your presentation. Remember. No volunteers, no show.

3)Light or heavy hands: Sit up. Place both arms towards the side. Left palm face up. Right palm face down. Shut your eyes. Your right wrist imagine that you are holding balloons made of helium and they are gently pulling your arm up and to the top. In your left hand, imagine a pile of heavy books, pulling your arm downwards and down. Add more balloons in your right hand, pulling it upwards (make your voice feel light and singing). Add additional books in your left hand making it feel heavier , and drag the hand back down (make your voice less pronounced and slow). After a few repetitions, you'll notice that your hands will show some vertical space. Ask your participants to look up and check out how much distance is between their hands.

4.) Stuck Hands 4) Stuck Hands (this is best done for a test on your own or a demonstration) to rest their hands against an even surface. For instance, a wall, table or even a bar for example. Explain to them that you've placed a super-strong adhesive on their hands and it is setting and sticking the hand on the wall. Similar to as before, repeat the words of being stuck in a firm manner and then test that the victim is not able to lift their hand off the surface. It is possible to extend this by asking them to pull their hand using a different hand, and then inform them that the second hand is stuck to the first. If you walk over to them and tell them they are free to move their hands as long as you let it happen.

5.) The Locked Arm Request your subject to extend an arm straight and form the fist. Inform them that your arm is becoming stiff as a steel bar. Remember how indestructible an iron bar can be. Like before, repeat the important phrases until you're certain they're paying you complete attention. Then, as before, make them examine their physical condition. They won't be in a position to bend their arm until you grant them permission, which is.

Inductions should be nothing more than telling the victim that they'll enter a trance state or hypnosis state, an utterly relaxed and open-minded state of mind (whatever it is you want to label it to satisfy legal or personal reasons) by saying'sleep and you tell them to sleep. Your true skill lies by adding some drama, for example, the trick of getting them to lie to their backs (stand behind them, gentle stroke of your finger across their forehead to yourself) by gently tapping their forehead, then placing your shoulder on their back and then gently (gently) pushing them forward by shaking their hands and pushing them toward the forward direction (again without violence) and then saying in a loud voice that you want them to go to sleep. Every induction is an adaptation on the idea of pre-planning and the command. It's your choice how you present it to your viewers. Take a look at Robert Temple's See-Saw Induction as a novel twist.

It is not necessary to push your victims around in any way that is incredibly forceful. They may be suffering from old (or recently) injuries that can be aggravated if you abruptly start pulling or pushing the victim around, therefore it is recommended to consult with them before you do so. The purpose of this sudden movements is to trigger some shock or surprise in order that your request to go to sleep is slipped in and accepted while the mind is contemplating the shock that the body just experienced.

Start by using a deepener as soon when they are tranced out. Encourage them to ease their arms, let loose the grip. Inform them that they're at a standing position or stand straight, not slide off of their chairs (as is appropriate) and they're doing fine. The"deepener" should be only repeating "Go deeper further and more" as well as repeating feeling of calm. Make sure that they're safe and steady before moving for the person next, if you're working in as a group.

Chapter 7: Hypnosis 101: What is Hypnosis and the Most Common Myths about Hypnosis

Hypnosis is an approach to tap into the nervous system, brain, and other body resources through controlled techniques, with the aim of helping you overcome negative behaviors and address specific psychosomatic issues. The practice of hypnosis is the ability to reduce distractions, improve responsiveness and increase your focus, and frequently as a way to other treatments.

Hypnosis is accomplished by utilizing procedures that allow one to achieve the state of hypnosis. The process of hypnosis puts the subconscious in the center of attention because it is by accessing unconscious that full power and effectiveness of hypnosis are revealed.

Hypnosis can be achieved by the practice of meditation as well as relaxation. In fact, the advancement of science and the realm of psycho and medical sciences has recognized that hypnosis can be an effective method to help patients and people suffering from problems with their behavior to overcome their difficulties or to handle them efficiently. However, even the fact that hypnosis has been used for a considerable time, a lot of people consider it a shady practice. Some people are unaware of the practice, while others are ignorant or dismiss the practice as a sort of spiritual or occult.

A lot of misconceptions about hypnosis stop individuals from benefiting from this effective therapeutic method. Let's look at a few of the myths that you and others have encountered.

Myths and Common Sense about Hypnosis

One of the biggest challenges that any innovative idea has to face is the propagation of myths. Since hypnosis isn't an entirely new concept there is a good chance that the number of myths people have created around it is endless. Here we will examine some of the most popular myths that have developed around the concept of hypnosis. Certain of them appear as being completely absurd at first glance however, believe me when I say there are those that still hold to these myths.

It is important to note there are myths that has stopped many from using this beneficial free-of-cost tool that anyone can benefit from to improve their lives. So, take a look at these myths with a view to dispel the myths surrounding hypnosis, and allowing it to everyone those who need it. It is very costly to be ignorant.

Myth: The Hollywood Films Effect

There are many movies you have seen from Hollywood or other places. Hypnosis is usually presented as a peculiar thing that people were born with. These characters are portrayed as a bit odd and capable of performing extraordinary things. They are usually depicted as mystical and controlling abilities.

The truth is that hypnosis isn't an inherent trait in humans. It is a method that allows every human being in order to harness their minds to their fullest extent. Hypnosis is a method to help you achieve what is feasible within the limits of human capability.

Myths: Hypnotists control what you say and how you feel, and make you perform actions you'd prefer not to do.

Truth: In the process of creating hypnosis the client is the one in control of the actions they take or do not do. They determine which suggestions to take into consideration and what suggestions to dismiss. A skilled hypnotist won't make you do something or making any statement. In reality, when you've been hypnotized, your enter a state of awareness and alertness and it becomes impossible to do anything without recognizing it. It is a popular belief that people don't know the state of the world around them during a hypnotic state. This is a myth that should be dismissed as a myth , too.

Myth: You can Easily Uncover Secrets Involuntary

Truth: This is another myth that is often repeated. While a skilled hypnotist may assist you in recalling events that you have experienced in the past However, the choice to reveal all details rests with the individual. As we've mentioned previously this process brings to an more alertness. It's impossible to do anything you're not aware of or to act in a reflexive manner. Keep in mind that the entire procedure is about managing your thoughts. What you think about or share is yours to decide. You can't be considered to be in control of your thoughts when you share details without consciously.

Myth: Hypnosis is intended for people with weak minds.

The fact is that hypnosis requires the sameness. It is not possible to do it on those with weak mental capabilities. In fact, hypnosis demands the ability to think clearly. Individuals with an IQ higher than average are perfect for the treatment since they can see and execute the process without any glitches. Hypnosis is not for a inexperienced mind or the foolish. Contrary to what many believe, this is the truth. Hypnosis is a skill that requires a highly educated and a strong mind.

Myth: You could be trapped in the trance

The fact that you're in a state of Trance doesn't mean you're not awake. If the hypnotist ceased talking then you'd feel a sense of alertness and then easily look up to verify that everything is working as planned. Many people are able to slip into a brief nap following which they awake completely aware of the world around them and feel at ease and relaxed.

Myth: Hypnosis can be dangerous

The truth is that it's false, except for two instances. As long that the client is in an area that is secure and safe there is absolutely no risk. I must make a usual disclaimer however. Hypnosis isn't advised for patients with epilepsy. If performed, the epileptic patient's body enters the state of complete relaxation. This hypnotic state can cause to the victim to experience epileptic seizures. Thus, epileptics aren't suitable for hypnosis.

Furthermore, do not attempt to use the art of hypnosis when working on machinery or driving. It is possible to slip into a trance , and result in harm to yourself or other people. Make sure that you are in a safe, secure space that is and free of any activity prior to start the hypnosis process. Hypnosis isn't just brainwashing. It is possible to revisit previous beliefs and ideas whenever they want. You are able to recall and think rationally even after hypnosis treatments.

Myth The occult practice of hypnosis includes hypnosis.

Truth: Hypnosis is a professional discipline that employs proven methods to get outcomes. In reality, hypnosis is not a religion-based practice in its practice, or its source.

The reason for neutrality has resulted in its acceptance by a variety of religions around the world as a powerful tool for treating various ailments that are that are related to thought and mental state. One of the numerous religions that have adopted it includes one of them being the Catholic Church.

Mythology: Hypnosis is a form of witchcraft

The fact is that hypnosis is a field of study that employs techniques that are scientifically developed to perform processes. The results can be tested and can be in direct or indirect ways affected by a variety of variables. Furthermore, hypnosis is focused on the positive results that the client will achieve. It doesn't make use of bizarre or nebulous objects or invoking any supernatural powers that are not part of the human mind. There are no charms , or props to create dramatic effect. In addition, you are able to do hypnosis wherever you want.

Myth that hypnosis is selective

The truth is that hypnosis isn't specific. Anyone is at ease. All that is needed is your willingness and availability. Modern guided hypnosis is now possible on the internet, with the effectiveness of the hypnosis determined by the person who is being the subject of the hypnosis. Nobody is innately destined to perform the art of hypnosis. It is a learned skill and anyone is able to learn about it and benefit from its numerous benefits

Myth: Hypnosis does not make you healthy

Fact: The reverse of the myth above is also true. Hypnosis is widely utilized to improve well-being and health. It helps alleviate people suffering from such ailments like depression, stress as well as anxiety, tinnitus, and many more. It can also be used to treat conditions such as arthritis and high blood Pressure.

Myth: You sleep during hypnosis

The truth is that you are in a state that is more awareness during the process of hypnosis.

Myth: You might become addicted or dependent on the hypnotist you have chosen to use

The truth is that hypnosis is designed to make you self-sufficient. It is intended to let you control your thoughts after the completion of a successful hypnosis session. Dependency is one of the main issues that hypnosis therapy can help to address.

Myth: If don't hear an hypnotist, it means you're not hypnotized.

In reality, hypnosis involves the hypnotist communicating with the person who is the client. The client is supposed to respond to the suggestions made by the person who is hypnotizing. It's an unnecessary waste of time to suggest things to someone who isn't able to hear the suggestions.

After we have debunked the most common myths about hypnosis and misconceptions, let's take a look at the ways you can get into an hypnosis-like state.

Chapter 8: The Hypnotic Environment

You should have the proper location to enhance the effects and experiences of self-hypnosis. The space itself must be comfortable (a few degrees higher than the ambient temperature is ideal) and the décor must be conducive to relaxing. The furniture, walls and rugs, the drapes, and floors should not be an obstruction.

Odors must also be eliminated. Plants do not pose the issue as long as you enjoy incense or other scents, absolutely make them available. However, you must eliminate any unpleasant or unpleasant smells.

If you're using the technique of eye fixation ensure that the object is not higher than the sofa or chair which you are relaxing on. Many patients enjoy doing their self-hypnosis while lying in couch or in their bed on the couch. Recliners are a better option. The subconscious mind has been programmed to think of lying down as sleeping. So if you're physically exhausted, you could easily get sleepy. Recliners don't possess that connection and might be more suitable to your physique.

A lot of people prefer to light candles of white in their self-hypnosis space. The room must be as peaceful as it can be. Shut the door and notify others present to not disrupt you for at least 30 minutes. It is advised to wear headphones when recording audio tracks. The headphones block out any sound and focus your hypnotist's voice into the subconscious mind of the subject. Other suggestions for your hypnosis area include:

1. Make sure you have a blanket close by.

2. Be sure to have tissues on hand.

3. Set up the recording device close to your location if you're planning to capture your experience.

4. A metronome, or a variety of metronome beats can be an ideal background for creating an illusion of hypnosis. It also assists in pacing your voice.

Recording your own music

It's initially apparent that making your own self-hypnosis recordings is a requirement for expertise and time that you might not have. This also implies an expensive procedure that might be over your budget. Actually, this is not the case.

You might be familiar with the commercially recorded self-hypnosis recordings. They are cheap and permit you to test this technique at the ease and in the privacy in the privacy of your home. Commercial recordings are great for your first exposure to self-hypnosis. However it's far better to create yourself recordings. You can make them personal to your personal goals. It's similar to buying a customized suit , rather than one that is available off the rack.

On average you will only need about an hour to create a top-quality self-hypnosis recording. It is also possible to learn more about the science and art of hypnosis when you make the recordings of your own.

There are just three easy steps to make your own recording of self-hypnosis. The first is the introduction into the state of hypnosis. It could be a common one of the numerous examples I provide in the subsequent chapters. Specific goals scripts are the second step. Finally, tips for getting up make up the third and last step. They are also available in the later chapters.

When recording, talk clearly and slowly. You might find it beneficial to play relaxing background music when recording. The background music could be used to block out any unwanted sounds - like traffic or voices from an adjacent room. Ocean waves or gentle rain spring in the countryside are easily accessible on the internet. Another option is to use a metronome , or the ticking of a clock to pacify your voice, and assist in stimulation into an euphoria.

If you listen to your self-hypnosis recordings you'll literally use the subconscious to create your future. Self-hypnosis is the term used to describe the building process by yourself. You don't have a middleman since clients and hypnotists are one in the same. When you use self-hypnosis, you're always in control since you are the one who gives the suggestions and directing the entire procedure. You are using your mind more effectively and using it in a private positive manner. Self-hypnosis is an educational and growth experience. It serves as a platform for positive changes.

You will be able to affirm your intention and objectives when you offer yourself positive suggestions for hypnosis. The practice will accelerate the process and help you improve your self-hypnosis skills. Practice with visualization exercises to help make these dreams real. Think of this as a chance to change old challenges into new ones.

The best time to do self-hypnosis is during the early morning, right after waking. You could be someone who sleeps, or you will experience energy peaking during the afternoon. Whatever your biological rhythm one thing you do not would like to do is surrender to the normal, but unproductive tendency to put off work. Self-hypnosis can be used during other times of the day when you need to unwind and concentrate on your goals.

If you use an existing script that are provided or creating a custom script from scratch, take note of these suggestions right after your usual introduction. Depending on the pace you take and the timeframe you pick the final recording should take about 1 1/2 hours long. You can record this every day, either once or twice over the course of a month. Do not record any more that 30 mins.

Success can happen anytime. It could happen instantly or you may experience it later. Minor changes are usually noticed within a few days, while significant changes can be observed within a couple of weeks. Some people are quick to respond to the messages in their recording, while other slow and slowly alter and develop incrementally every day. Over time, you'll build up your confidence and be able to write yourself scripts.

These are a few additional suggestions to help you make more effective use of your recordings:

1. If you are about for a state Are your fingers showing indications of curling? Are your hands tight? Are they tight? If yes allow your hands to uncurl and loosen your hands. Are your legs crossed? Crossing them is a good way to improve circulation. Are there areas of your shoes or clothing that are tight? Let them loose for your individual convenience. Relax to a certain extent.

2. If you would like to be more active role in the recording session put yourself in an armchair or bed and lay down after the recording session has ended.

3. To use your recording in the evening don't include a wake-up segment. Just suggest that you fall straight into your sleep cycle, waking up from the state of hypnosis.

4. It's quite normal for your mind to wander in self-hypnosis. Be aware that you are inefficient during this time. It is possible to experience the state of hypnoamnesia. This is the presence of a significant amount of the hypnosis. The activities of your conscious mind and/or level of boredom are irrelevant to the self-hypnosis you use. We are concerned with the subconscious.

5. It is strongly advised to include music in space-free during the recordings. This will increase your Trance experience and block distracting ambient sounds.

6. After you have recorded your script, include an alarm clock. The phrase "wake-up" isn't correct, as you're never truly asleep or in a state of unconscious. The term "wake-up" is utilized because it's so that it is a part of the perception of the concept of hypnosis. The aim of the wake-up segment is to help your mind to

gradually adjust its attention to the present world.

The following script is a good starting point to record your first video. This is an easy exercise that includes an induction component and a wake-up feature:

(Ocean can be heard in the background for around 10 seconds before the metronome beats behind to match your voice)

"Sit in a comfortable position and listen to the metronome's rhythm as you listen to the background music. Each beat will make you feel more relaxed.

"Listen when I count backwards, from one. Each backwards count will get each muscle in your body so relaxed that by the number 1 it will put you in a profound and relaxed state of the hypnosis.

20th, 29th, 18th deep at peace, completely relaxed.

"17, 16, 15, down, down, down.

"14 13", 13, 12 Very deeply.

"11 10, 9 9", deeply, totally at ease.

"Eight, seven, six, so very sleepy. Five four, three deeply at peace, completely calm. Two, one sleepy. 20-20-20.

"You are currently in a tense state of relaxation. Pay attention as I count backwards, but this time, from 7 to 1. When I begin counting in reverse from 7 to 1 you'll hear the metronome's beats on the background diminish in volume, and then decrease in volume each time until I get to the number of one. At that it will be silent other than my voice. You will be at a comfortable and deep state of sleep."

(Decrease beats of the metronome until count is one, and then they're gone)

"Seven, deeper, deeper, deeper, down, down, down.

"Six, deeper, deeper, deeper, down, down, down.

"Five, deeper, deeper, deeper, down, down, down,

"Four, deeper, deeper, deeper, down, down, down.

"Three, deeper, deeper, deeper, down, down, down.

"Two, deeper, deeper, deeper, down, down, down.

"One deep, deeply relaxed, completely asleep. 20-20-20.

"You are now in a tense state of relaxation and hypnosis. Repeating the number 20 three times through your voice will get you in this wonderful deep state of hypnosis fast and extremely deeply. This will bring you there quicker and more deeply every time you attempt self-hypnosis."

(You may add any instructions you like to add from now on and finish the trance by following:)

"Now just the next few seconds ... as I count five ... you'll awake and will be awake. You'll feel much better after this restful and refreshing sleep. You'll feel totally at peace ... mentally and physically. physically and mentally ... completely serene and calm ... without even the any feeling of sleepiness or fatigue.

"And the next this time ... you'll not only be able to drift to sleep quicker and more easily ... But you'll be able to be able to sleep more deeply.

"One ... Two ... Three ... Four ... Five ... alert and rejuvenated."

Chapter 9: What Is It?

To "Be Hypnotized?"

As well as an altered state of mind, it is an actual process. The process is an natural procedure that is designed to get you into a state of concentrated awareness where your mind is more open to positive suggestions understanding, insight, and awareness. In this state of focus that you are able to quickly integrate new abilities strategies, strategies, strengths and knowledge, as well as eliminate negative thoughts, emotions and routines.

With your permission, consent and desire an experienced hypnosis professional can assist you in taking charge of the life you live, especially in areas that you've felt out of control.

Take back control of the unproductive, unwanted and unneeded thoughts, feelings and habits that hinder you from creating the life you've always wanted.

The only thing you need to meet to be hypnotized are consent and a desire. When you're engaged in self-hypnosis, or working with a professional, granting yourself permission to engage in the procedure, and having an intention to experience it aligns with your desired outcomes throughout and following the session is all you require to do in order to be hypnotized. It's all you require to experience the benefits completely.

It's similar to the conscious decision we make whenever we decide to watch a film. No matter whether we're watching the film in a theatre or sitting in the comforts at home prior to starting the film, we've taken the decision to suspend our disbelief.

As if a small portion of us had not already taken the decision to suspend disbelief and at least subconsciously realize that we've accepted our consent and have a want to "go through the motions" and fully experience the emotions and experiences the film might bring and we wouldn't be able to ignore the fact that we're watching actors in characters in a script written by someone else, and used speaking to cameras on a set that has been made up for a film that is set.

When we have that agreement or desire we become a part of the film and we are able to experience all the feelings that actors and directors, producers, musicians and cinematographers have led us towards.

We love the process and its results as well as the similar thing can happen in the event that you want to be controlled. An unforgettable experience that can have the potential to change your life!

What is it like to feel

To be to be hypnotized?

Because hypnosis is an experience that is different for everyone there's no one experience that everyone has. However, there are a variety of common emotions and experiences shared by all people who experience hypnosis.

Many report feeling calm and at ease. You might notice that it feels as if you're in your favourite chair after a long day. Many people find themselves in a relaxed state of mind while in hypnosis such as relaxing in a hammock while enjoying your well-deserved beach holiday.

Some feel a profound sensation of calm, which has them feeling a heavy weight throughout their body as if they could not raise their arms, legs or even the eyelids even when they wanted to.

Some people report that the relaxation is a blissful sensation of light and floating as if they're floating in the air in the chair they're in.

It's also not uncommon to not experience anything distinctive or unique during the entire session, instead you're in a chair in a quiet room listening to a conversation.

These diverse experiences occur due to the fact that hypnosis isn't just about your body or the sensations you're feeling, but the state of your mind or the thoughts you're processing deep in your unconscious mind.

When you go through hypnosis, you might feel diverse sensations at different intervals, and even during one session. There may be a strong feeling of comfort in your legs, arms or even your body as if you're in a comfortable position you're. There may be a slight floating sensation like you're floating above the spot. It might feel as if you're lying in bed or sitting in awe of every word spoken.

You may also find your thoughts drifting off and wandering away from words you're hearing to another place or thoughts.

All is normal and okay. Everything you feel is okay, since there's no single hypnotized sensation that you can pinpoint.

In actual fact, during the hypnosis session, if you want to move or scratch, swallow or change your position, you are at ease to do it. It will allow you relax more.

At times, you'll be aware of everything going on around you , and obviously, you should never give the capability to process and think. react and respond in whatever way you think is appropriate.

Actually, the majority of people believe that they aren't in a hypnosis , or that they're not doing anything wrong, since they're still thinking, observing and observing. There's a chance that you're your mind wandering over what you'll need to accomplish later... contemplating if the sound was caused by your stomach getting a little rumbling, or professional hypnotists... in which case your hand is reclining... perhaps any other thought that wander between your head. This is perfectly normal. Your conscious mind is doing what the conscious mind is doing - noticing and being conscious.

Incredibly, even though being in deeper trance is amazing it is only a slight level of trance is needed to allow the work to be accomplished. It is not uncommon to prefer the experiences physically as well as mentally experienced by those in deep states of trance. It allows us to truly "check out" and have a little mental vacation. But it's not necessary to changes. It's usually something that happens through the practice of it, but it's not an absolute requirement.

Chapter 10: The Three Keys To Effective Use of Hypnosis

If you're working with a Hypnotherapist or self-hypnosis there are three pillars to the success of the power of hypnosis. These are self-motivationand repetition, and real or credible suggestions.

1. The motivation for change must be derived from within.

You've already heard this.

It is a fact that regardless of how much you think that someone else is in need of change, no matter how much you wish for them to change, you are unable to influence them to change. This is also true for you. The motivation to change should come from within you.

For instance, let's say you're trying to change your lifestyle because someone else is trying to convince you to shed weight or quit smoking. It's not going to be effective. I've had the pleasure of working with many clients who wish to lose weight or stop smoking. They sought me out because their doctor or spouse suggested they change. They don't do well with hypnosis.

On the other hand people who visit because they have a goal in mind and are looking to stop smoking cigarettes or lose weight typically react quickly and quickly.

Therefore, prior to beginning using hypnosis to help you on your personal improvement journey first, you must determine the things you'd like to change and the reason you'd like the change to take place within your mind. A clear and consistent intention to change will assist in helping the suggestions of hypnosis to take root and be incorporated into your daily life. If you're having trouble understanding this then you should consult an experienced hypnotherapist to assist you in completing this process more swiftly.

2. Repeat, repeat, and repeat.

It is essential to keep going for it in nearly everything you do. For instance, if you would like to improve the level of fitness you have, don't expect to hit the gym for a few minutes and achieve the level of fitness you want. You'll need to exercise every day for the rest of your life. Similar to the use of hypnosis. To do it effectively, it requires regular repetition, at a minimum when you are forming the new habits that will empower you.

Be aware that your actions are simple habits, something you've developed gradually as time passes. It's fascinating to realize that the majority of behaviors aren't "on" or "off," but happen or "are triggers" because of different kinds of stimuli. Sometimes, triggers can be triggered by an assortment of circumstances or events. This means that you could visit a hypnotist the same day with a set of triggers you want to be worked on, and feel at ease when you leave however, the next day, when you're exposed to new set of triggers you will experience the same symptoms repeatedly.

It's good to know that that you had one trigger in control. To change your routines it is necessary to work on the triggers that are not addressed. This could take a few sessions to be ironed out, which is the reason that many hypnotherapists offer self-hypnosis audio recordings for you to listen to at home.

3. The suggestions should be realistic or plausible.

The third element that can be crucial for effective use of hypnosis for personal transformation is that the suggestions you receive must be believable or realistic. Your mind won't take a suggestion you don't or can't accept. Whatever the degree of certainty it seems or the positive it could be for you, before you take a decision you must first be able to accept it as a real possibility.

For instance telling a chocolate lover that chocolate is unpleasant to them and make them sick is a difficult for their minds to comprehend. If such a notion was to be implemented it will only last just a short period of time since it would be astonishment to anyone who is a true chocolate enthusiast.

In these situations one of the most effective strategies I've tried is that when you eat chocolate, it's not going to taste as delicious as it did before. This is much more realistic and credible, which is why it's accepted by the majority of people. After a certain amount of repetition (remember the second key point) over a long period over time, it loses a lot of its appeal, and ultimately decreases its power over the person.

Chapter 11: Preparing the Ground

Hypnotists are constantly hearing a person claim that they "was not hypnotized because ..."

To remove some of these annoying "becauses" Let's talk about some of the issues to understand what we've been experiencing.

Do I lose consciousness?

Whatever way you get hypnotized, you'll never be able to lose consciousness. If you've ever woken in the night to use the bathroom and later claimed next day that they did not recall doing it had (a) been able to transition between sleep and hypnosis, and (b) suffered mild amnesia and never noticed it.

Hypnosis is essentially a replica of the natural sleep but it's a little different since under hypnosis you could be able to observe your self-recorded "sleep". Some patients have been known to say that "I noticed myself in my sleep."

Don't think that you will lose consciousness, or to disappear beyond the realm of possibility or experience an amazing extraordinary or bizarre situation.

The notion that you are being lost of consciousness is often propagated through Stage Hypnosis programs (nowadays being a hot topic on television). Consider this: the stage hypnotist informs the subject that "He is in the Tropics in the Tropics, where it's 100 degrees" and ...", the person, who everybody believes that he is "asleep" starts to sweat and then remove his coat. It is likely that he "heard" that suggestion, so he was not sleeping. He was hypnotized, but he wasn't asleep.

It is a state of mind that occurs when your conscious brain is disengaged, resulting in an imitation of sleep, yet the conscious mind remains as an eyewitness to the whole process. Therefore, don't expect to sleep, even if you're under the influence of hypnosis. Expect to experience the state of complete relaxation and reliving the physical aspects of sleep, However, you will not be asleep.

Why was my mind wandering?

When you are in hypnosis, your brain probably will be wandering as it is normal for your mind to wander, this wandering is simply the sub-vocal association of thoughts that is often referred to as thinking. If you notice that your mind wanders in your exercise routine, just allow it to wander.

Maybe I was trying to for too long?

The answer to this question was already given just a few thousand years back: "Who amongst you, could increase his stature by one inch with your will?"

Any amount of determination to do, of trying to do something, of trying to help yourself towards getting to the point of each exercise will aid you in any way. Actually the more you attempt more, the less likely you are to achieve. Only "trying" you can expect of you is to test and maintain your routine.

If you're looking to prove your self that there is no way to achieve a desired result, or to answer the question to yourself once and all, this "pencil test" will help you.

Place one of your pencils between your right thumb and your index finger. Keep the pencil in place and then say to yourself mentally: "I want to drop this pencil."

You can repeat that statement until the end of the world and still find it difficult to drop the pencil. To drop it first, you have to change your mind to "I will be dropping the pencil."

Training yourself to self Hypnosis

Before we start our journey, we'll begin by getting ready for the process of being hypnotized. In this regard, I've created an exercise set of four to be performed during this week.

Body Postures

Two postures are described and illustrated to help you in your daily practice of conditioning exercises and then later for your regular sessions of hypnosis. These are the positions that will give you the most effective results since they reduce the amount of external stimulation.

These exercises should ideally done in a quiet space and in dim lighting to reduce any possibility of disturbances.

All clothing items that are tight as well as other obstructions to freedom of movement (glasses belts, belts, girdles and tie, wristwatch etc.).) are to be untightened or removed.

Sleeping on the mattress

A few days of practicing is enough for you to determine which posture is best for you. If you opt for the lying down position, you should lie on your back, your legs relaxed and slightly separated to ensure that your feet create an open 'V'. A gentle support on the knees' back like a folded mattress sheet or pillow can help you achieve the most relaxation for your legs. Your knees shouldn't touch. Find the most comfortable place for the shoulders and head by trying different methods of helping them.

The arms should be stretched along with the body, and are loose and at ease. The fingers should be separated and shouldn't contact the body.

Sitting down

The exercises could be performed from a sitting position with the condition of taking note of some anatomical and physiological aspects.

Pick a chair that has either a reclining back or straightback chair, based on your own personal preferences.

Its back reclining chair must be tall enough to allow the head to be supported when it sits comfortably. The fingers and hands should be resting on the armrests of the chair or better yet hanging off to the side of the chair. You can even put hands on lap if want to.

The legs must be parallel, while the thighs form an angle of about a half. The feet are placed directly on the floor and the edges of the chair should not put pressure too heavily on the back of the knees or the thighs. of knees.

The standard sitting chair is the most common type of chair used since it allows one to exercise at any time and from any location.

In short, choose the position where you are comfortable enough to lie down.

The key is in your hands.

This course will assist you develop self-hypnosis and all the benefits that it brings when you follow the guidelines provided.

There's no number of books you read or rereading you can do to prevent you from doing the tests - and even being able to pass them.

In order to purchase anything particularly a brand new psychotherapy facility, the appropriate cost must be paid.

The price here is the consistent and diligent practice of conditioning exercises for the next five days. One method of getting over the resistance is to set the duration (about twenty to forty minutes) over the next five days you will be able to practice these exercises. In normal conditions you will be able to achieve an acceptable level of self-hypnosis in this period. (Some people might want to keep their exercises for conditioning for several more weeks. The more they are conditioned to perform the procedure the better results they will be able to expect.

Your Schedule

Here is a list of 4 exercises to build up your conditioning. Do each one for the next five days.

The purpose

The goal in these exercise is teach your body to follow your thinking. For example, if you imagine that "My hands are weighty," your hands should be able to feel heavy. This is the foundation of all hypnotic techniques and it is therefore essential to master at this point.

The exercise must be completed before the next one.

Each exercise in this section is terminated through repeating 3 times: "Everything is normal." Following each termination of a particular exercise, you will be required to stroll around for approximately 1 minute.

And you're prepared for the next workout. This way of ending the exercise has the following goals:

1. Remove the residual effects of the previous exercise.

2. Be sure to assure yourself that, if you practice the exercise that you're not gaining from the exercise.

The energy of the preceding exercise.

EXERCISE ONE

Aim:

Instant relaxation of the muscles in the arms and nearby muscles repeating five times the following sentence: "Both my arms are as heavy as lead."

Ten times per minute - without eyes shut - and one final sentence: "Everything is normal."

The five sentences that must follow are

1. My left arm seems very heavy.

2. The arm I have on my right is extremely heavy.

3. My right arm seems very heavy.

4. The left side of my arm weighs extremely heavy.

5. My arms are both as heavy as lead.

(If you are occupied by the minutiae of counting the number of times you've completed the sentences, you can use this strategy:

One of my arms is very heavy.

Two My right arm is very heavy.

Three Right arm of mine is massive.

- - - - and the list goes on and on until you reach 10 times, and then you move on until the next sentence, continuing in the same manner.)

When you repeat these phrases as you sit there, you are thinking about your arms, starting from your fingertips to your shoulders. Imagine the muscles as employees that are able to take orders from your mind.

Procedure:

1. Put yourself into the the position you want to be in.

2. Take 3 slow, steady breaths.

3. Shut your eyes. 4. Repeat each of the five sentences 10 times.

5. Repetition the sentence in your mind three times.

6. Stand up, stretch your muscles and walk around to relieve yourself of the negative effects of

exercise. 7. Repeat the steps 1 and 2.

8. Recite the sentence mentally: "Both my arms are heavy as lead." Five times.

Repeat this exercise until you feel instant and total relief and weightlessness in your arms by repeating the phrase five times. In normal conditions it will take between 3 and 4 repetitions.

EXERCISE TWO

AIM:

The instant relaxation of muscles of the legs and those around them by repeating five times the following sentence: "Both my legs are heavier than lead."

Ten times per second while keeping your eyes closed and one

Final sentence: "Everything is normal." The five sentences that must repeat are

1. The right side of my leg feels very heavy.

2. My left leg feels quite heavy.

3. The left side of my leg feels a bit heavy.

4. The left side of my leg feels quite heavy.

5. Both of my legs weigh as much due to lead.

When you repeat these phrases and think about your legs from the tips of your feet all the way to your legs. The muscles could be thought of to be your employees , who follow your thoughts. They have only two things: be tight and taut, or let loose and limp.

Procedure:

1. Put yourself into the position you prefer.

2. Take 3 slow, steady breaths.

3. Shut your eyes.

4. Repeat each of the five sentences 10 times.

5. Repetition the sentence in your mind three times.

6. Stretch yourself, get up and walk around to release yourself from the consequences of exercise.

7. Repeat the steps One and Two. 8. Recite the sentence mentally: "Both my legs are heavier than lead." Five times.

Repeat this process until you feel instant and total ease and lightness in your legs. Repeat the above phrase five times. In normal conditions it is recommended to take 3-4 repetitions.

Exercise THREE

AIM:

The instant and automatic closing of the eyes using five times the phrase: "My eyes are closed tightly."

Method:

Mechanical repetition of five sentences at ten times each while closed eyes - and of one final sentence: "Everything is normal."

The five sentences that need to repeat are

1. My eyelids are full.

2. My eyelids are extremely heavy.

3. My eyelids weigh as much like lead.

4. Eyes are shutting.

5. My eyes are tightly closed.

As you repeat these phrases while you think about your eyes, becoming heavier and heavier as you repeat the sentences above. Imagine two tiny magnets, with opposite polarity, that are glued to the upper and lower lids of each eye , pulling against one another.

Procedure:

1. Put yourself into the the position of your choice. 2. Take 3 slow, steady breaths.

3. Take your eyes off the screen.

4. Repeat each of the five sentences 10 times.

5. Repetition the sentence in your mind three times.

6. Take a step up, stretch your muscles and move around to get rid of the effects of exercise.

7. Repeat the steps 1 and 2.

8. Recite the sentence mentally: "My eyes are closed and my eyes are closed." Five times.

Repeat this practice until you feel an instantaneous and immediate closing of your eyes. Repeat the sentence above five times. In normal conditions it could take 3-4 repetitions.

EXERCISE FOUR

AIM:

A state of hypnosis that is light with five times the sentence: "My whole body is more hefty with each breath."

Method:

Mechanical repetition of four sentences in the different versions 10 times each with eyes closed of one

Final sentence "Everything happens as normal." The four sentences to be repeated are:

1. My legs are both as heavier than lead.

2. Both of my legs weigh as much due to lead.

3. My eyes are tightly closed.

4. My entire body gets more hefty with each breath.

When you repeat these words while you think about your legs, arms and eyes, which become heavier and heavier as you repeat the above phrases.

Procedure:

1. Place yourself in the the position of your choice.

2. Take 3 slow, steady breaths.

3. Shut your eyes. 4. Repetition the sentences 10 times.

5. Repetition the sentence in your mind three times.

6. Stretch yourself, get up and walk around in order to relieve yourself of the effects of exercising.

7. Repeat the steps one and two.

8. Repeat the sentence mentally: "My whole body is more heaver with each breath." Five times.

Repeat this exercise until you feel complete and immediate relaxation and weightlessness in your legs and arms, as well as the an automatic closing of your eyes by repeating the previous sentence five times.

In normal conditions it should take 3-4 repetitions.

Chapter 12: Hypnosuggestive Study Techniques In Psychotherapy As Well as Psychological Assistance

To treat people suffering from alcoholism, we have employed a methods, such as the "coding" developed by AR Dovzhenko. The essence of the method is in the development of a persistent psychological framework for abstinence from alcohol. It is made possible by applying various psychotherapeutic methods and strategies that are triggered through stress factors, which aim to increase the instinct for self-protection (in specific). The approach is implemented throughout the phases. The first stage is creating and strengthening, the implementation of treatment and definitely the result is positive. It uses indirect suggestion. In the second phase, comes into play the urge of self-defense, which is reflected in as a "cult of character" doctor. Group sessions were held using various psychotherapeutic methods which were performed against the backdrop of gipnoidnyh state. In the forefront, rational psychotherapy. According to Dovzhenko eliminating the person's desire to combat drinking can lead to the elimination of the desire for alcohol. The patients are instructed that physician's referral efforts are stable. concentration of stimulation of neurons within the brain that block the urge to drink for long periods. The third stage (actually the coding) can take between 2 and 3 minutes and is an essential recommendation.

The use of hypnosis as well as the neurotic gipnoanaliza is a highly effective technique which reduces the time spent in psychoanalysis. Gipnoanaliz blends hypnosis and cathartic techniques, psychoanalysis, and so on. The patient is usually taught to rapidly enter the state of hypnosis. Then, it is used for analysis of free association hypnosis such as vnushonnye dreaming, regression of age and so on.

Another kind of hypnosuggestive techniques for application - the development of creative skills. Effects of trance on creativity and ability to discover Bowers (1967), Krippner (1968) and other. The results of the research showed that the freedom of people from the consequences of the protective effects of daily routine life (fear of criticism and attachment to the status quo and unpredictability) during a state of an hypnotic trance can increase the creative potential of . Soviet researchers (V. O. Raykov and Tihomirov) were also able to conduct similar tests, and the results showed that the emergence of creativity through hypnosis depends on the condition and perception of the person to whom the subject is portrayed.

One of the many uses for Hypnosis was one of one of the most effective methods for therapy of pain. Hypnosis, for the first time to be used for pain treatment, was employed by London doctor Elliotson during the first half in the late 19th century. In the beginning of the twenty-first century J. Esdaille, who was working in India and India, underwent thousands of minor surgeries and more than three hundred severe surgeries under the influence of hypnosis.

Over the next few years in the following years, particularly following the discovery and development the effectiveness of anesthesia, it was discovered that hypnosis was employed during the ever-so-rare surgical procedure. Its use was mostly in surgery wards was a part of the preparation of patients for surgery. The purpose of this procedure is to ease anxiety, stress and fear of surgery and the repercussions. Based on the patient's suggestibility, it can reduce the use of analgesics administered and speeds the recovery.

Recently, hypnotherapy is being used to treat migraine and its more drug-resistant forms of treatment. Some doctors have seen complete cure in 30-45 percent of cases. Those who decrease the frequency and pain of attacks, but they still have about 25-30 percentage of patients. The most effective results were achieved with self-hypnosis and autokontsentratsii.

In certain countries, hypnosis has been widely used to help with labor pain. The result of hypnosis was Koroleva Elizaveta.

Hypnosis can bring about positive outcomes for women who suffer from issues related to the stressors of home life. They are prone to stress and anxiety. Women experience changes in their ovarian cycle between who are between 45 and 50 years old due to the lack of sexual hormone Estrin however, the symptoms that accompany these changes are neurological origins (pain and irritation, the rush in blood flow to the brain, depression cancerophobia). All of these conditions can be cured quickly with the aid of an hypnosis session.

In the US Hypnosis is utilized to remove teeth and to alleviate anxiety about visiting the dentist. In the case of ongoing cases, hypnosis is used to decrease the fear of complications that can result from long-term therapy with drugs.

Hypnosis is effective for the treatment of ghost pain. Patients who have undergone amputations over the years were suffering from excruciating pain in the limbs that were never there. The pain can be unbearable and not respond to the use of drugs. One Finnish surgeon treated dozens of similar patients, and got excellent results in 60 percent of cases. They did this by allowing the patient was immersed in a in a state of hypnosis.

It has helped for managing hypertension, reducing the stress that comes with the high pressure. It also helps in the treatment of conditions related to the digestive tract (vomiting gastric spasms, esophageal spasms, stomach and intestinal cramps, constipation, etc.). Hypnosis is a proven method of treatment for psychosomatic conditions like gastric ulcer and asthma bronchial.

Through hypnosis, you can use it to treat itching and warts, allergic lesions. Positive results were achieved through by hypnosis, as well as motor-related disorders (convulsions and speech disorders, tics, and many more.).

Hypnosis has proven effective to treat sexual problems, including in frigidity and impotence. In the maintenance therapy, hypnosis can be utilized to combat the addiction to nicotine, alcohol and tobacco and other substances to treat addiction to drugs. The application of this method to lose weight.

J. Slade (1995 pp. 30-31) says that hypnosis it is possible to combat diverse dependencies, and they are viewed as trauma. This is similar to the reprogramming of your hard drive of your computer, when you think of the human mind as being a computer and its psyche as the drive. Slade is a hypnotist that has been quoted "I employ a new form of hypnosis which produces an instant result. It means that the client doesn't feel any discomfort due to "lag" like, for instance food, an issue that can occurs with other methods that rely solely on Will ... It is quite simple to get rid of the desire to smoke , by injecting into the mind of the patient. It is easy, effectiveand its outcomes are long-lasting. The dialogue that the mind has with itself it's a conversation between an 8 year old child, therefore I make use of very simple phrases and thoughts. I sketch the images into the mind of the patient, and as my patient's in an hypnotic state, the patient is aware of the words I'm using. "

It should be noted that this is an hypnosis technique that is specifically designed for patients who are suffering from trauma, because alcoholism and smoking are believed to cause harm. This type of addiction will eventually cause death for many, is a fact. Rosenhan and Seligman claim that "when tabagism hypnosis is utilized to connect smoking to the imagination of adversivnogo content." This method can result in the first restriction on smoking. However, follow-up studies over time reveal a significant rate of the recurrence.

Particularly important is the use of hypnosis for cases of multiple personalities. The treatment procedure in this situation is very difficult. The initial stage is determined by the patient's awareness of the issue. While for a long time his condition was a baffling stateof mind, having amnesia I have heard from other patients concerning his strange behavior. The patient does not necessarily have to realize that it has multiple personality types. The doctor hypnotizes the patient creating an alter ego, and lets them freely speak. The patient is also instructed to listen, and later it appears to stay alive personalities. The patient is asked to recall everything she was through when taken out of the hypnotic state. The realization of the existence of other people can cause immense anxiety and stress. However, it is essential that the patient maintains the realization of who they are. If you do this, you might encounter one of the toughest difficulties: the patient might become ill again and fall into a condition of autism, thereby avoiding any confrontation with reality. This can be very uncomfortable for the patient. In this situation the therapist needs to contact the patients.

It is important to note that in the field of psychiatry, the use of hypnosis is still used to fight anxiety, phobias and anxiety. It can also be used to treat insomnia disorders, memory, and attention. Hypnotherapy is distinguished by the constant development of improvements techniques.

Hypnosis is generally viewed as one of the ties to the whole treatment system , in combination with other techniques. It is based on conditioned reactions, psychoanalysis, anger management and many more.

Based on the type of illness and the patient who is able to provide individual or group therapy. The strain relief that comes from the hypnosis, it is more readily accepted as a suggestions for therapy, there is the possibility of an interaction with the therapist that has more confidence.

Hypnosis is a method used in experimental psychology. The majority of the research has been conducted to determine the possibility that hypnosis can have an impact on the physiological reactions of blood supply system the digestive, respiratory system, and many other. Hypnosis as well as related methods (e.g. techniques to relax) are employed to aid in different areas in psychology (e.g. sports psychology, for instance.).

In the writings by authors of Japan, Germany, the former Soviet Union and other countries We find data on the effects of hypnosis in conjunction with self-control, as well as other suggestions to deal with the extreme anxiety in sporting events, the improvement of certain sports techniques to maximize your physical and mental reserves to prepare for competitions and finally in order to lessen or even total relief from discomfort.

Alongside self-hypnosis, hypnosis is also utilized, which can be used to reduce the vulnerability to stress, improve self-esteem, decrease weight, stop smoking, eliminate anxiety and fears and treat psychosomatic illnesses and decrease the pain (Mizioiek 1996, s. 30,).

It is important to note that hypnosis works for treating mental and physical pain. However, it is advised that the legitimacy of the application of hypnosis is based on a myriad of psychological, medical and ethical factors that can be summarized as follows: following guidelines:

The rights to perform the hypnotherapy procedure is only granted to those who are certified and ethically perfected complexion.

The introduction into a hypnotic trance and hold sessions hypnotic only is possible with the consent of the patient.

Hypnotherapeutic and hypnotherapeutic treatments are a way to restore physical and mental well-being. In this regard, those who have the ability to utilize therapeutic Hypnosis is the sole right of doctors and psychologists.

Hypnosis is not allowed to improve vision and patient faith.

There is no basis to interfere with the practice of hypnotherapy that is in the patient's privacy or moral responsibilities.

People who are involved in hypnotherapy for suffering should be systematically enhancing their psychological and medical knowledge.

By adhering to the principles, you can ensure the reliability of the application of the hypnosis. However, it is important to keep in mind that hypnosis an unanswered question in the psychological and medical sense.

Ericksonian Hypnosis

The use of suggestive methods in teaching

Hypnosis and suggestions are utilized in the active learning process, incorporating components of relaxing, suggestion , and games the an immersion technique. This is a method of learning that gives the pupil with an inner sense of liberation, and reveals the possibilities of a person. The immersion method can be used particularly when you are learning a new language. It is a way to bypass the conventional notion of training as a hard job and, by employing various suggestions and suggestions, it helps build confidence in their capabilities and helps in the transition from formal training to self-training.

Please consider "dive" that we can find in R.M.Granovskoy. The word "immersion" she interprets as "active learning approach that incorporates relaxation elements, suggestion and play" in which case the words "immersion" along with "suggestopediya" they are synonymous. She points out that contrary to other methods of training, mainly founded on a lack of conviction "immersion method is heavily dependent on suggestion." It is important to remember it is "suggestion (or suggestions) is a process that has an impact on the psychic sphere of the person with less awareness and a lack of awareness and implementation of the content, and the absence of active and purposeful understanding that uses logical analysis and assessment in relation to prior experience and to the condition that the person is in. " In the wake of suggestion R.M.Granovskaya is astonished by the high level of attention and gains (liberation) the ability to think creatively. "Immersion method is built on three pillars which are the enjoyment and relaxation within the class, and the interplay of the subconscious and conscious communication, and the two-way interaction in the process of learning."

As these concepts have been formulated by R.M.Granovskoy G.K.Lozanova and refined themby referring to the source:

"The concept of" happiness and a relaxed "should be recognized to the extent of that it is psevdopassivnosti behaviour in relation to learning. It is essential to manage an external student, who maintains the stress and keeps the mind, as well as its internal setting for studying. Lax and joy do not take away the stage, as well as the ongoing process of studying.

The principle of unity of consciousness' and the concept of nesoznavaniya "requires the participation of an organized holistic persona as well as her conscious and unwitting roles.

The concept that follows from "suggestive relationship" guides the learning process by activating each reserve. This principle demands continuous updates about the outcomes of learning. " According to G.K.Lozanov states, the entire set of principles should be in indivisible unification and at all times of the learning process being that is carried out simultaneously. The application of these rules can be accomplished by using three kinds of methods which are: A) psychological and b) educational as well as) artistic.

"Psychological agents regulate the perception of peripheral stimuli and emotions and are geared towards the application of motivational complexes as well as system settings and in general, require stimulation by the person." Nespitsificheskaya the students' mental responsiveness developed a specific situation exercise. According to her R.M.Granovskaya components include the following: a) the solemnity of the moment; b) the prestige of the teacher and their credibility and credibility; c) the performance of the band members; g) accessibility of students. When we look at"immersion" in "immersion" of the group in T.N.Smirnovoy we find that "the effectiveness of the training process depends on the cooperation of groups. This is achievable only when there is a high degree of respect and goodwill. Training participants should sit in semicircles thus ensuring seeing each group of students. In the event that there are handful of light sources, the instructor can alter the amount of illumination. " Additionally, the efficacy of the training is a factor in the convenience of seating, being insulated from noise outside.

Regarding teachers' authority his presence is essential to the effective application of suggestopedii. It is without authority that any authority to make suggestions. "Where confidence is present, there's not necessarily evidence. Trust in the students' expertise and skills of the teacher can boost their confidence in their ability to absorb education materials and, consequently will be extremely helpful to the overall improvement in their capacity to think and cognitive ability. " "Authority is a source of expectation and higher impact of suggestions." It is important to note that the assistance should be uplifting rather than restrictive and restricting power of.

At present, suggestive strategies are employed in the game. Through vnushonnogo, sleep relaxation occurs and efficiency recuperation faster than an extended vacation during the wake state. Autogenic and hypnosis-based training has been proven to be a successful way to overcome adverse conditions prior to launch. Vnushonny sleep-rest is suggested as a method of reducing mental and psychological stress for a variety of mental and physical conditions faced by athletes.

Fear is the most deadly among all feelings. The extensive research and images that are dedicated to fear, provide the ideal foundation for deeper understanding of this crucial emotion. Literature on the subject has grown slightly. However, the issue of fear among students in junior classes is very popular currently. The issue of fear is rarely discussed in the daily routine of school. In the end, it all started when school started to be introduced that there were associated fears that children began to experience. So, even in kindergarten, students have to pass the tests for anxiety and overcome the fear barrier within their minds.

Psychologists have identified two methods to reduce anxiety in children.

The development of constructive behavior in stressful situations for children, and mastering strategies that help cope with the stress, fear, and excitement.

Building self-confidence, enhancing self-esteem and beliefs about themselves, and concern about "personal development" for man.

In these circumstances that we can offer suggestions for ways to proceed.

The principle idea behind the Ericsson the hypnosis

Milton Erickson was born in the log cabin of the small town of mining within the Western US in 1901. Through his entire life, Milton Erickson practiced trance. The state was later referred to as "Ericksonian Hypnosis." Methods, concepts and techniques that were developed from Erickson are now beginning to take over modern psychotherapy.

Erickson was able to come up with ideas and invent, since it was required in states that were not common to ordinary people. Erikson born in the year 1898 was devoid of the sensation of color. Erikson was unable to differentiate between sounds of their height or in a position to play the tune. When he was a kid, he was diagnosed with dyslexia (disturbance of reading). When he was 17, he experienced an outbreak of polio. He fully recovered thanks to having just recently developed rehabilitation program. At 51, the man was struck by the disease again, but this time, he was able to recover a little. In the last 10 years, he was in the wheelchair. He was constantly in pain and the condition was partly crippled. He was completely paralyzed in his tongue and the right hand.

Sometimes, with the vigor of people, these limitations can be a source of by the creativity of Erickson. He was able to recognize opportunities and appreciate the capacity of all human beings.

If there is another term that is hypnotic trance, it's the state wherein consciousness is changed, that is not the same as normal to enter into a trance with Erickson wasn't difficult. Erickson could explain his view that he had experienced to his patient. The patient, in an effort to comprehend it, tried to see the world around him and, in the end the condition altered his consciousness. He entered an hypnotic state.

As an undergraduate teacher at the school of Milton Erickson carefully studied the writings from A. R. Luriya who was a specialist in hypnosis as well as the word association tests. This knowledge was tested with his own hands, attempting to develop something that was more refined from what was already available. In 1936, he published an article that described what he learned from his tests with the test of word association. The test's examples are the following. Man will provide the stimulus for any of that describes his issue. He's conscious that he won't. In this instance the stimulant term "stomach" Test subject used the following phrases"large, anxiety baby, fear surgery disease, forgetting. Then, it was about her unwanted pregnancythat she couldn't recall. By using a reverse logic Erickson realized his therapist was able to take care of for the entire procedure and deliver an email to the patient disguised as an actual story. This is when he came up with the idea of developing his own language of hypnosis in which the suggestion is delivered in a gentle, non-violent manner and without affecting the patient's awareness. The language are poetry imagery, imagery, a range of information provided to the unconscious and conscious mindfully and in accordance with the wishes of the patient.

Chapter 13: Self Hypnosis Techniques

#Imagery

Imagery is a form of visualization, which is the process of creating images in your head with your imagination. It could also encompass all senses, including as well as smell, taste sound , and sight. While the majority of people utilize their visual senses most of the time however, to make the visualization efficient, it is necessary to include all of the aspects of other senses. The self-hypnosis mental image can be worth many pages of verbal advice. You can develop your own personal image by combining your personal memories and experiences so that you can strengthen your ideas. Here are some exercises that you can try to improve your ability to visualize:

You can imagine someone you know including yourself, and imagine their distinctive characteristics.

Take a close look at the object, then shut your eyes while trying to imagine it.

Visualize your living space by switching from one room room. Then, take a moment to imagine what tastes, smells, sounds and appears to be like.

There are two main ways to use imagery to help you achieve your desired goal:

Process images

It is imagining the steps or steps you must follow to reach the goals you desire. For example, a footballer could imagine scoring the perfect goal when he gets close to the goal line.

Result imagery

The visualization creates visual images that depict the desired goal or desired outcome as if it's been achieved. For

149

instance, if are required to give a speech to your coworkers, you may imagine yourself giving the speech confidently, receiving applause following you have delivered the message, as well as also the positive outcome of your impressive speech.

Research has demonstrated that the act of visualizing can create subtle, but tangible changes in the muscles involved with the imagined activity. When you repeat the task repeatedly in your head the subconscious mind creates the memories of an action that was successfully completed and it is then trained to achieve the result you wish to attain.

Let's suppose that you wish to shed weight. The result images can help you imagine yourself at the ideal weight and size that you would like to be. In the mirror, and visualize yourself as slim and thin as you would like, and fit perfectly in the dress or suit you'd like. Imagine the feeling you'd have having achieved your target. It is also possible to use process imagery to imagine you eating smaller and smaller portion sizes of your food. Additionally it is possible to create a more precise picture by picturing yourself taking food items on your plate when you are satisfied. This will help increase the positive steps you'll be taking to accomplish your goals. The ability to visualize and imagine is largely dependent on the unconscious mind. To be successful with images, you have to become as inventive and imaginative as you are able to. Make use of your personal memories and experiences to add flavors and smells, textures sound, colors, and sounds to be as captivating and real as they can.

#The Hypnotic Language

Every person has their own personal collection of memories and memories. And you are able to communicate with yourself in the language that has special meaning for you, based on the experiences you've had. Your subconscious mind is more prone to ideas that reflect the world you live in. It is more likely that you will succeed with self-hypnosis when you employ your own personal symbols and words when you make suggestions. You should try to discover the predominant method of communication, which is the meaning you are most acquaint to, and then employ words and phrases that are connected to that specific feeling in your personal self-hypnosis language.

For instance, if it's visually-based, then you can say "I can see" ...", or"I can see." If it's an auditory language, then you can say "I hear it" ..."," or "it is like". If it's the Kinaesthetic language, then you could say "it is like" ..."... and like that. Research has shown the likelihood that people follow your hypnotic thoughts more effectively if they match your personal style of communication.

Symbols are basically images are used to symbolize something else. You can incorporate them into your thoughts to show the goals you wish to attain. For example, falling leaves off the trees may be a sign of surrendering to problems and clouds glistening in the blue sky could be a sign of a peaceful attitude. Furthermore, these symbols will more likely influence on your thoughts if you are able to draw inspiration from your own personal experiences as your subconscious is more likely to be able to relate to these symbols.

As a guideline, before you begin your self-hypnosis sessions ensure you've planned your goals and come up with appropriate symbols and images that can help you achieve the goals. Make use of your own memory to create images try to make them as creative and imaginative as you can when explaining them. Make your ideas concrete and feasible. You're less likely to make decisions based on vague images or descriptions. The ability to articulate the same concept in different ways increases the likelihood of being successful. Also, you should try to make your suggestions positive rather than negative. People generally respond negatively to negative suggestions. We do not like being given the message "NO". However an idea that is constructed positively that has a positive outcome will be more likely to get a positive response. For example, if, for instance, you say to yourself that you don't consume chocolate any more it is interpreted as an order to be negative which you are likely to reject or ignore.

Include emotive phrases in your suggestions. Positive emotions can help in strengthening your ideas. For example, "I breathe effortlessly ..." or "I feel incredibly at ease". Be sure to avoid making your story unbalanced or unreal Try to reach a high-quality target, then create it to perfection.

#Breathing Exercises, Relaxation And Relaxation

A deep breath is an tried and tested method to relax completely. This is an old technique that yoga instructors enjoy using and is extremely useful and enjoyable when used in self-hypnosis. In general, your everyday breathing is typically rapid and shallow, and usually involves contraction and expansion that of your chest. In contrast deep diaphragmatic breathing can be much more beneficial and is derived in the abdominal. This breathing style allows you to stretch your stomach outwards when you inhale. This eventually draws the diaphragmatic membrane beneath your lungs, allowing your lungs to take in air and fill the space. Inhale slowly with your nose, exhale slowly with your mouth. This slow deep, continuous breathing triggers an energizing response within your body that is the opposite of the adrenaline-prone "fight or fight or flight" response.

Relaxation can have numerous benefits, such as muscular relaxation as well as an increase in blood flow to the extremities, as well as a reduction in heart rate.

A breathing exercise

Begin by taking the deep breath diaphragmatically as you breathe in through your nostrils, and count up three times with your lungs fully. Take a deep breath through the mouth for 6 counts. Take four seconds to rest before repeating the exercise. Keep your mind calm and calm while breathing. But do not inhale so much until your lungs begin to burn or hurt. If you are feeling lightheaded or dizzy in a certain point it is possible to rest for a moment before moving on.

It is possible to practice this breathing practice anywhere and at any time. You can use it to reduce tension or pressure. You can take 5 deep and slow breaths as you prepare yourself for self-hypnosis.

#Progressive relaxation

It is a method of relaxation, which was created by the psychologist Edmund Jacobson. It simply involves focusing on the various muscles in your body, in isolation and gradually through the sequence, and then relaxing any tension between those muscles. Edmund developed this method on the assumption that it's impossible for a mind that is anxious to be a part of a relaxed body. It is important to apply a particular amount of tension to the muscles of your face, shoulders and necks as these muscles tend to be prone to holding lots of tension.

The technique involves tensing the muscles while breathing into them, allowing the breath to remain in your lungs for a couple of seconds, and then exhaling slowly and slowly to let go of all tension completely. It is possible to do this for specific muscle groups until your entire body is at ease. The main muscle groups that can relax using this method are your legs, hands as well as feet, arms with the head and face buttocks, stomach, the neck, chest and back shoulders.

The process of passive progressive relaxation is identical to the previous active progressive relaxation. However, it does not need you to tighten your muscles in a vigorous manner. Instead, you just imagine the tension draining through your body as you exhale and inhale while progressively working your body. You can further enhance the experience by picturing tension as a fluid draining from your body when you breathe. This is an extremely simple and relaxed technique of self-hypnosis and relaxation that can be done practically anyplace.

Once you're at peace, consider what it feels like, and make a mental image that portrays your state of relaxation.

#Relaxation Technique

Choose an object that is suitable and fixate your eyes on it. maintain it above your eye level, without any obstruction. Watch your eyelids become droopy and then breathe deeply.

Imagine the object through your mind's perspective and let it sink deeper into your subconscious mind. Count slowly, not more than 10. Then say "I am calming".

As you feel tired Imagine yourself in a trance. Set a goal for yourself and set out to reach it.

Let your mind absorb the positive energy. To break out of the Trance, begin counting backwards.

#Age Regressive Technique

Think about the past and imagine your timeline. Think about all the moments that are a an integral part of your life.

Make a sudden switch in which you imagine your future along similar line.

159

Take advantage of your dreams for the future.

Visualize a long track of where you are at the moment. Keep your focus and fight against the difficulties of today.

Imagine walking forward towards the your future after overcoming all obstacles. Look for the point at which you are victorious.

*To get out of trance yourself returning to your current date and time.

Hand Levitation Technique (For alleviating the pain)

*Place your palms on your lap, then gaze downwards.

*Words are firmly pointing towards your hands, and then fix your eyes on a specific area.

Imagine hands becoming lighter in weight, and then rising like the shape of a balloon. This will cause your hand to rise up.

Let your hand move up. Your eyes remain fixed on the fixed spot.

Imagine your hand touching the part of your body that is hurting. The area could involve your arm, leg or face. It could also be your tooth.

*Let your hand rest on the injured area and take in the discomfort.

Feel your hand gently sucking up all the pain until you feel relaxed.

Gradually get out of the trance by counting from 10 to 1 in reverse.

#Talk-to- Yourself Technique

Relax yourself and prepare to speak to yourself to hypnotize yourself. Relax and center your mind.

Relax your body and loosen your shoulders and spine. Consider that your body melts and softens.

Imagine your mind standing in front of your face and begin to talk to it. Discuss problems that require to be solved. It should also be relaxed and soothing to ensure that the you get the desired result.

*To get out of Trance, tell your mind to return and follow you.#Goal Setting Method (for setting new goals or habits)

Think of two types of wires passing through each nerve in your body. One wire is responsible for the body's voluntary functions and the other handles involuntary functions.

Use your index finger as an electrical switch to control the two wires. At present, the switch is on.

Now, slowly close your eyes and relax your body. Relieve your stress by releasing your index finger to turn off the.

Relax your body and mind like its strength is gone. Imagine you are implementing an entirely new habit or a goal.

162

*Multiply your positive and encouraging feelings to make it appear as if you're an accomplished person.

Each day, follow these steps in 20-minute increments.

To come out of the Trance, take a deep breath and then snap your fingers back.

#Mind Programming Technique

Find a private and serene space and lie down with your eyes closed. Begin to imagine how you'd conduct your life should you be given the option.

Leave your past behind and be in charge of your life in the future. Do your best to separate yourself from the past.

You can imagine yourself as the cockpit of a plane, and as pilot flying through the air and avoiding clouds that are dark in the sky.

Treat the stormy and dark clouds as obstacles in your life slowing your advancement. It could be a result of your own thoughts, experiences or even a few incidents.

Get past those dark clouds that are hindering your journey to enjoy an overall good spiritual, mental and physical health.

Allow your mind's subconscious to overcome these obstacles and be in a large and comfortable space.

Repeat the visualization procedure until you feel more comfortable.

#Creating Imbalance Technique

*Arrange for a rocking seat and sit down on it with a gentle touch.

Begin to rock yourself until your head feels slightly dizzy. It will eventually relax your mind and you will begin to enjoy the experience.

Close your eyes and picture your entire body reacting to the vibrations. In time, you'll be in Trance.

164

Allow your brain to comprehend the goal you are aiming for by speaking loudly to yourself.

Keep rocking yourself until your wish to stay in a trance. If you're ready to come out then slow down the movement in the seat.

Do not stop the rocking of the chair abruptly in case you be suffering from severe headaches.

"Shocking" your Nervous System Technique

The self-hypnosis method requires you to use a the ability to speak with authority and force to shock your nervous system.

Get into the trance you desire in a pleasant way. Find a technique that will take you effortlessly into trance.

Keep your surroundings quiet and shut your eyes for a while before you start jolting yourself. Keep yourself prepared by preparing a powerful and quick command that will put your brain at a high alert. It could be a specific command, or even a heal command that can assist you achieve your goal.

Now shout the command loudly to obtain a quick and intense sensation. There is a chance that you will be able to come out of the trance in this moment. To prevent this from happening take a moment to allow yourself to be deeper into the state of trance. In this moment your mind will be in a trance state and will follow commands to condition it in the right way.

You can get out of trance simply by lying down for a period of period of time while keeping your eyes shut. You'll snap out of the trance when the impact of your loud commands is diminished.

The process of hypnotizing yourself can be difficult which is why you could have to employ certain strategies to face some of the difficulties that you'll face like difficulties in achieving an euphoric state. Here are some suggestions for positive phrases that you can use in order to help make your experience simpler. Before we proceed we'll take a brief look at the steps to test your the hypnotic trance.

Chapter 14: Helping Through Hypnosis

If you've been following all the tips I've given so far, and you have been working consistently, you may have witnessed the incredible effects of hypnosis on your own. In this way, you're likely to want to share your newly acquired skills with anyone who could benefit from help. Before you convince someone of accepting the hypnotic trick on them, I would recommend that you think about some things to consider as a precautions. In addition, I'll briefly discuss the ethics involved in using hypnosis to influence an individual.

First, let me remind you that the only way to hypnotize yourself is through self-hypnosis. Particularly, one needs to desire to be hypnotized before they can do it in order to be hypnotized, regardless of the reason. The purpose of a hypnotist is to assist in making a person feel hypnotized and then giving the appropriate suggestions. Being hypnotized implies that you exert your efforts and concentrate on creating the whole process and allowing yourself to be relaxed. You should be obvious that you are not able to alter the free will of a person or be in conflict with their values and convictions. So, the first principle to be aware of when using hypnosis to one is to never give advice that is contrary to an individual's goal. They will be aware of this and quit participating, and there's a good chance that they won't be able to trust you again.

Second, I'd like to remind you of the rules of conduct listed in chapter 3. If you don't get trained and be certified as a hypnotherapist never attempt to hypnotize any person suffering from physical or mental health issues, or those who are going through difficulties with their relationships, and do not go through an individual's memory bank. This could result in potentially dangerous outcomes you do not wish to bear the burden of. So, how could a aspiring hypnotist do to aid in the process? My suggestion is to keep it simple. It is possible to help someone in your family to quit smoking, learn the art of calming their nerves during difficult situations or alleviate pain when they get tattoos. The most common rule of thumb is that if a physician is not required then you are able to assist. The process of using hypnosis to help someone are identical to those for self-hypnosis that are described in chapters 3 and 4. The distinction is that instead of putting yourself in an euphoric state and then giving instructions for guiding an individual into that state.

Find an open-minded participant who would like to be attracted to. This is a given and you shouldn't attempt to trick someone just to show you are capable of it. Most importantly, do not attempt to influence or trick individuals into agreeing to be hypnotized. You're already in breach of what is morally acceptable! The most important thing to consider before using hypnosis on someone - or requesting someone to hypnotize you or even hypnotizing someone else is the creation of trust between them.

Once you've identified a suitable participant make sure you review these basic steps with the person you are going to begin:

• Inform them of what they can be prepared for. Your client may have misconceptions about hypnosis. You can alleviate their anxieties and fears by providing them with an overview of what hypnosis actually is and not. Define how they'll fall when they're put into the trance, using your personal experience of self-hypnosis. They'll be more open once their minds are relaxed.

Are they hypnotized previously? If they've had experience being hypnotized ask them the reason for it what they felt at the time, how the experience was like, what advice they received and what resulted. This will help you comprehend how hypnotizable they're and what they'll respond to.

What goals are they trying to accomplish with the use of hypnosis? Do they want to get to get a better sleep? To reduce anxiety and stress? To achieve your weight-loss goals? Chat it over with your hypnosis companion to discuss solutions, and then use the information to come up with a solution.

After you've gone over all the fundamentals and have your script in place, locate the time to be at a calm pace and eliminate any distractions. When your partner is prepared and you are able to proceed by bringing about hypnosis and giving the suggestion in chapters 3 and 4.

As opposed to performing self-hypnosis the moment you instruct an individual to fall under, you may choose to remain quiet for a couple of minutes and then let them absorb the suggestions or explain to them the things they need to imagine after entering the suggestions in a verbal form. This will be contingent on what your client is comfortable withand it is something you will work out with them, possibly involving some trial and error. If you're guiding your subject to create a creative visualization, be sure to ask your participant to engage all of their senses. Therefore, aside from telling them "You imagine yourself doing that," ....", and describing the things they'd be able to smell, hear, touch and taste. Don't simply paint the whole picture, but also transport them to another location and time. Once you've finished you can gently take them out of the trance using an exaggerated suggestion to wake them up.

When your subject is able to come out from a trance, engage in an open post-hypnosis dialogue about the experience. Ask the subject how they feel, and receive feedback on how you performed as an person who hypnotizes. Are they willing to let themselves be hypnotized once more by you? Do they have suggestions for how you can help them? They may have suggestions of hypnotic scripts they'd like to test. Make sure you note these ideas in your log.

Take a look at the Good Stuff

What is the best way to develop yourself than to teach others? You're not only doing them a favor through teaching them an valuable ability they can utilize to improve their own lives, but you will also be able to learn from them and improve your own skills as you go along. If you're looking to test your skills at hypnotizing other people maybe you'd like to think about partnering with someone who is also interested in mastering the art and can serve as your hypnosis companion. After you've succeeded in hypnotizing on the subject, ask them to do the same next time. Learning to hypnotize yourself is enjoyable and rewarding however, it's much more fun with someone to study with!

A Dark Face of Hypnosis

While you explore how to hypnotize, and make use of it to improve your life, and other people, I'd like to highlight a dark aspect that I believe everyone who has attempted to master the field should know about. I'm talking about using hypnosis in entertainment as well as other purposes that are shady.

Let's begin with one that most of us are familiar with the stage hypnosis. In 2015 the Stage hypnosis Chris Jones appeared on the talent show America's Got Talent. Judge Howie Mandel was able to agree to be controlled by Jones in the performance. Mandel is afflicted with the most severe germaphobia because of the condition known as Obsessive Compulsion Disorder (OCD) and is notorious for his refusal to shake hands with judges. Jones amazed the audience with his captivating Mandel and making the talented judge shake hands with him as well as three other judges. Jones offered Mandel the impression that everyone was wearing a thin, latex glove which are not noticeable (which there isn't any). After watching the replay, Mandel was mortified and openly admitted to going to therapy following the incident.

If Mandel been the hypnotherapist, it would be convinced that human hand is not something to be scared of, and that they aren't pantry dishes that harbour germs because his mental illness had led him to be unable to rationally fear. It could have taken just only a couple of sessions of hypnotherapy in order to cure Mandel of his disorder by removing layers of fear that were irrational, instead of fooling his brain into believing that all around him was wearing gloves that were invisible until he is released from the state of trance.

The skeptical would say that stage hypnosis is fake, staged to entertain, and claim that both the hypnotist as well as "volunteer" were in a symbiosis. It's not far from the reality. There are stage shows that hypnotize that are set up completely. There are also people like Jones who do hypnosis in the stage, without manipulation for the sake of entertainment.

A stage hypnotist will choose their audience from the ones that are the most hypnotizable. They accomplish this by giving the audience a test for suggestibility with a brief introduction, and then a short suggestion to identify those who respond to a simple suggestion using the language of permissive. In the event, for example, as the hypnotist enters the stage, they'll request the audience to shut their eyes and then say something like, "You can close your eyes right now. Just close your eyes and pay attention to me. Your eyelids will be closed and stay shut because they're too heavy to lift. If you are unable to lift your eyelids, the more weighty you'll feel them and the more they'll remain closed." If they notice those in the audience that aren't able in opening their eyes they will be able to determine who to call on the stage.

Is stage hypnosis dangerous? Many hypnotists, both clinical and academic, believe so. They don't care about the health and safety of their audience members and are more focused on getting a reaction from their audience. In contrast to healthcare professionals who employ the use of hypnosis as part of their clinical practice and therapists on stage, stage hypnotists do not carefully formulate their suggestions in a way that's suitable and safe for the person who is participating. If you visit a clinical hypnotherapist, it is likely that you are informed upfront the kind of advice you will be given prior to being controlled. When you are hypnotized by a stage hypnotist you're in their hands at the point you are willing to be hypnotized. The worst part is that this type of hypnosis is used to perpetuate the negative perceptions regarding the art, which means people who are exposed to it are scared and do not appreciate the numerous benefits that the art of hypnosis offers.

But there's more! There's a darker application of hypnosis, where hypnotists employ coercive techniques to induce victims to agree to be hypnotized by them. This is the method employed by psychopaths who seek to maintain their victims' attachment to them, prior to when they get into the cycle of abuse and control. They'll carefully choose those who are emotionally vulnerable, and then continue to woo their victims by smothering the victim with love and affection. Slowly, they would make up scenarios to win the trust and cooperation of the person before putting them into the state of trance that they're unaware they have agreed to.

It is important to know about the various forms of hypnosis available to avoid being a reluctant participant and, obviously, refrain from attempting them yourself. Once you're equipped with knowledge of how hypnosis works, then you are able to defend yourself by identifying the hypnotic language. Do not follow the flimsy instructions or surrender to the hypnotic language of permissive. If someone starts an exchange with you and then utters random phrases like "Allow yourself to relax," ...", Be on the watch and alert them for their ploy! The use of hypnosis is only for entertainment or to harm other people. You don't know the extent of harm you're doing.

Leave the Kids Alone

Hypnosis is usually a non-invasive and safe method of treatment to anyone no matter what age. If you are a hypnotist who is just beginning but, don't try to hypnotize children younger than 13. If you think it's harmless and safe, why not utilize your newly acquired abilities to help an individual child who is having difficulty learning, or to convince them to stop from biting their nails? I would strongly suggest against doing it.

Children do not have the ability to participate in the practice of hypnosis. Because they lack the type of cognitive resistance adults do typically, children are significantly more susceptible to suggestions. You do not want to be creating something in the mind of a child that can cause a variety of problems later on. Additionally, a child could be suffering from a disorder which isn't a solution through the use of hypnosis. In the beginning of this chapter, I mentioned chapter that the first with hypnotic messages occurs through our parents. In reality, parents could have inadvertently hypnotized their children to believe that this world to be a risky area, or have produced enthusiastic and confident children. The power of words can be very effective to children's minds.

In the field of clinical hypnosis kids have successfully been treated to treat a variety of ailments, such as bedwetting temper tantrums and persistent nightmares. If you are aware of a child that you think might benefit from hypnosis visit an hypnotherapist so that they can be evaluated and treated. A hypnotherapist can also teach parents and guardians about hypnotic techniques and suggest ways to help children manage problems. Thus, you're better off letting your kids be the professionals.

It could be a breeze to train children to use one-line statements to self-affirm themselves, when they help them deal with the issue. For example, if a child is frequently upset about being called names at school, you can explain to them something like, "When people say things to you that make your unhappy, you'll not listen to them and move on." Do not attempt to place the child in a state of stupor on your own until you are properly trained.

Conclusion

Self-hypnosis is an innate state that humans can experience. It can be explained by saying that we all go into a state of trance that is light prior to falling to sleep. Self-hypnosis, whether with one form or another is a technique that has been used for a long the years. The benefits of self-hypnosis are therapeutic, relaxing as well as calming when it is practiced regularly and correctly.

Self-hypnosis is free of adverse effects and isn't injurious, so it can appeal to all people, regardless of beliefs or genders, as well as different walks of life. Furthermore, self-hypnosis is cheap and doesn't require any equipment to be carried out. So, anyone can learn to know self-hypnosis techniques and benefit from the this method.

The estimate is that two percent of people employ self-hypnosis, and receive amazing results using the method. This means that you are likely to be being among the growing amount of people who utilize self-hypnosis to achieve success on a principle. The extent of self-improvement and overall success of self-hypnosis will be restricted by the limitations you set for yourself.

www.ingramcontent.com/pod-product-compliance
Lightning Source LLC
Chambersburg PA
CBHW060329030426
42336CB00011B/1265